ROYAL HISTORICAL SOCIETY

STUDIES IN HISTORY

New Series

THE DYING AND THE DOCTORS

THE MEDICAL REVOLUTION IN SEVENTEENTH-CENTURY ENGLAND

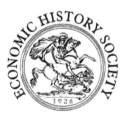
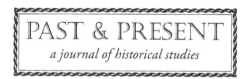

THE DYING AND THE DOCTORS

THE MEDICAL REVOLUTION IN SEVENTEENTH-CENTURY ENGLAND

Ian Mortimer

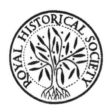

THE ROYAL HISTORICAL SOCIETY
THE BOYDELL PRESS

First published 2009
Paperback edition 2015

A Royal Historical Society publication
Published by The Boydell Press
an imprint of Boydell & Brewer Ltd
PO Box 9, Woodbridge, Suffolk IP12 3DF, UK
and of Boydell & Brewer Inc.
668 Mt Hope Avenue, Rochester, NY 14620–2731, USA
website: www.boydellandbrewer.com

ISBN 978 0 86193 302 0 hardback
ISBN 978 0 86193 326 6 paperback

ISSN 0269–2244

A CIP catalogue record for this book is available
from the British Library

THIS BOOK IS DEDICATED TO THREE SCHOLARS WHO HAVE
BEEN AS KIND AS THEY HAVE BEEN INSPIRING:
RALPH HOULBROOKE, MARGARET PELLING
AND JONATHAN BARRY

Contents

List of Figures

List of Tables

The publication of this book has been made possible by a grant
from The Scouloudi Foundation in association with the
Institute of Historical Research

Acknowledgements

My first and foremost debt of gratitude is to my wife, Sophie, who laboured under the weight of three children while I worked on this book. Without her support it probably would not have been started, and without her continued support it would certainly never have been completed.

I also owe a very significant debt to Dr Jonathan Barry (University of Exeter) and Dr Margaret Pelling (University of Oxford) for agreeing to take me on as a research student, and for their support thoughout my period of study and subsequently. I must also mention my gratitude to Professor Ralph Houlbrooke (University of Reading) who originally led me to probate accounts as a source during my stint as a Research Officer at Reading University in 1993–4. I am also very grateful to the anonymous peer referee who recommended publication, to Professor Mark Overton (University of Exeter) and to Christine Linehan who helped in the editorial process.

I am very grateful for financial support to the Arts and Humanities Research Board, the Wellcome Trust, the Newby Trust, the Royal Historical Society and the Joyce Youings Fund (administered by the University of Exeter).

I am grateful also to archivists around the country who responded to my detailed questions on probate accounts in their possession. I would especially like to thank staff at the county record offices of Berkshire (Reading), West Sussex (Chichester), Kent (Maidstone) and Wiltshire (Trowbridge). At Trowbridge, Mr Steven Hobbs was especially helpful in arranging access to the documents despite their being re-sorted, re-numbered and re-catalogued at the time of consultation. I also am grateful to staff at Devon Record Office, for allowing me to copy many of the diocesan licences in their keeping.

Finally, certain individuals have been very supportive, including Robert and Julie Mortimer, who allowed me to use their house as a base for research in Chichester; Andrew and Marina Wall for allowing me to use their house as a base for research in East Kent; and Zak Reddan and Mary Fawcett, for allowing me to stay while researching in London and for obtaining items from the Wellcome Trust Library on my behalf. To all these people I am very grateful.

Ian Mortimer

Abbreviations

BRO   Berkshire Record Office, Reading
CKS   Centre for Kentish Studies, Maidstone
DRO   Devon Record Office, Exeter
GEV   Gross Estate Value (the value of the moveable chattels of an estate with which the administrator charged himself. It normally corresponds with the total value of the inventory, but in some cases includes data not available to the inventory compilers)
WRO   Wiltshire and Swindon Record Office, Trowbridge
WSRO   West Sussex Record Office, Chichester

Note on the text

In quotations from primary sources
    {} denote deletions
    <> denote insertions into the text
All dates have been converted to historical years, i.e. with the new year at 1st January.
Undated documents have been dated to the most probable decade according to their archival context.

Introduction

If social history were a series of landscapes, then the most dramatic terrain – the steepest mountains – would be found in the social history of medicine. The problems posed by severe illnesses, incapacity and death have led to the most profound social developments, affecting almost every aspect of human life. The sixteenth and seventeenth centuries are particularly important in this respect, and cannot be regarded as simply the low foothills before the steeper slopes of modern medical discoveries. Indeed, with regard to the acceptance of the need for a high-quality, regulated medical profession, the three centuries before the Apothecaries Act of 1815 were the steep slopes. However, if we question what people actually did when they were seriously ill at any given time in this period, we run into problems. There is a dearth of primary source material for measuring change. As a consequence, the process whereby society became medicalised – in the sense that individuals regularly sought professional medical solutions to serious illnesses and ailments rather than spiritual or amateur nursing help – remains vague and relatively unexplored.

Most previous attempts to map out the process of medicalisation have either been narratives of one of the three main branches of the medical profession (physicians, surgeons and apothecaries) or studies of the symptoms of the change (examinations of the developing outlook on spiritual physic and religion, for example), not the change itself. Overviews of the subject have used diaries, practitioner casebooks and a wealth of other social material, but they have been vague as to whether the whole country experienced a shift of attitude or whether it was just London, or just the middling sort, who turned to medicine with greater frequency at the end of the seventeenth century. Some writers have developed detailed regional quantifications of death and linked these to outbreaks of illnesses, but no one has attempted to show similar links between death and medicine. The nearest to a quantification of the process of medicalisation has been the ongoing struggle to correlate the number of medical practitioners and the population in any given place at a given time, from the work of R. M. S. McConaghey, John Raach and R. S. Roberts in the early 1960s to the seminal article, 'Medical practitioners', by Margaret Pelling and Charles Webster, and Margaret Pelling's subsequent refinements of the statistics.[1] These snapshots in time cannot

---

[1] R. M. S. McConaghey, 'The history of rural medical practice', in F. N. L. Poynter (ed.), *The evolution of medical practice in Britain*, London 1961, 117–43; J. Raach, *A directory of English country physicians, 1603–43*, London 1962; R. S. Roberts, 'The personnel and practice of medicine in Tudor and Stuart England: part 1: the provinces', *Medical*

quantify the changes affecting society. Although categories of care have been diligently researched, the only full-scale attempts to map out the medical services available in a region according to patients' whereabouts and social status have been those based on the extensive papers of Richard Napier, especially Ronald Sawyer's study of him.[2] However, Sawyer's work was about just one man, and a highly unusual man at that, and therefore not only lacks regional variation but also the context of temporal change. When there were perhaps three or four thousand men practising medicine or surgery in some remunerative form or other in the early seventeenth century, Napier's career can hardly be considered illustrative of the whole medical profession.

One way to remedy this problem, and to conduct a thorough examination of the medicalisation of early modern society, lies in examining the collections of probate accounts which are to be found predominantly in the diocesan record offices of England. By examining as many accounts as possible to see what proportions of the dying purchased medical help in any particular decade, a model of medical involvement for that region can be constructed. This can be refined to differentiate between people of high or low status, or urban consumption in relation to rural. In this way, in theory, the level of medicalisation in 1600 can be compared with that in 1700 in any given place for which sufficient records survive, and for a variety of social classes. In short, it is possible to observe the pattern by which the English turned from praying for spiritual physic to paying for medicines when struggling with grave illnesses.

That is the theory. In practice the patterns of medicalisation can be reconstructed for only a small portion of the country. Probate accounts are by far the scarcest of the three main types of probate document: fewer than forty-three thousand survive (compared to two million wills and a million probate inventories).[3] Only five counties – Kent, Lincolnshire, Berkshire, Sussex and Wiltshire – have more than a thousand examples, permitting an analysis of each decade of the seventeenth century.[4] Any study based on probate accounts must therefore be centred largely on these counties. Nevertheless, the opportunity to reconstruct the medicalisation of any part of the country is one not to be missed, especially when it is possibly unique.

History vi (1962), 363–82; M. Pelling and C. Webster, 'Medical practitioners', in C. Webster (ed.), *Health, medicine and morality in the sixteenth century*, Cambridge 1979, 165–236; M. Pelling, 'Tradition and diversity: medical practice in Norwich, 1550–1640', in Instituto Nazionale de Studi sul Rinascimento, *Scienze credenze occulte livelli di cultura*, Florence 1982, 159–71.
[2] R. Sawyer, 'Patients, healers and disease in the south east Midlands, 1597–1634', unpubl. PhD diss. Wisconsin–Madison 1985.
[3] A. L. Erickson, 'Using probate accounts', in T. Arkell, N. Evans and N. Goose, *When death us do part*, Oxford 2000, 103–19 at p. 104.
[4] Ibid. 107.

What are probate accounts?

The 'probate account' is a convenient collective term used to describe the accounts created by executors and administrators in the course of administering a deceased person's estate. It is a product of the system by means of which the ecclesiastical courts supervised the administration of the estates of deceased men, spinsters and widows from the mid-sixteenth century until the eighteenth.[5] It was the last document drawn up in the process of administering the estate of a deceased person, meant to be a final drawing of a line beneath the process of administration.

The general pattern of creation may be summarised briefly. There are four identifiable periods: first, the period prior to about 1570, when the account was evolving into a recognisably standard form. Second, there is the period between the establishment of the form of the document, in about 1570, and the Interregnum, when the ecclesiastical courts were suspended. The third period, from 1660 to 1685, runs from the restoration of the ecclesiastical courts to the Act for the Reviving and Continuance of Several Acts of Parliament of 1685, which amplified the Act for the Better Settling of Intestates' Estates of 1670–1.[6] As a result of this act, accounts were only to be created at the instigation of a relative or creditor of the deceased. The final period, during which a comparatively small number of accounts were made, is the period after the 1685 act. Most counties have only a few documents after 1690, and Kent, the exception, has very few after 1720.

Virtually all the accounts surviving today are official copies drawn up for presentation in court. Accountants – as those who administered an estate and submitted an account were normally called – kept a record of expenditure which was later put into proper form by clerks, usually a year after the death of the deceased but sometimes after a longer period. The few extant drafts in existence show that the formal account was not a straightforward copy of a draft. Not only did a certain amount of polite tidying take place, but details were included in the account which are not in the drafts. Close examination of the draft accounts reveals that the additional details were obtained through an interrogative process, probably in an interview held for drawing up the formal account for presentation to the court.[7] Some draft accounts bear the clerk's scribbled notes and insertions as a result of

---

[5] A few executors' accounts are known from the Middle Ages, and the latest date from the nineteenth century. See *Berkshire probate accounts, 1573–1712*, ed. I. Mortimer (Berkshire Record Society iv, 1999), p. vii, and Erickson, 'Using probate accounts', 104.

[6] The crucial act is 1 James II, c. 17 (1685), which included the specific prohibition in the case of intestates for an administrator to be commanded to produce an account. The original act of 1670–1 (22 & 23 Charles II c. 10) was further clarified by the last clause in 29 Charles II c. 3 (preventing the law from applying to intestate married women): O. Ruffhead, *Statutes at large*, London 1786, iii. 334–5, 364, 388.

[7] I. Mortimer, 'Why were probate accounts made? Methodological issues concerning the historical use of administrators' and executors' accounts', *Archives* xxxi (2006), 4–5.

asking pertinent questions. Most accounts carry the entry 'for conceaving of this accompt in writing and Counsell about the same', probably referring to the dialogue between the accountant and the clerk.[8] From this it may be seen that the surviving formal probate accounts are products of a process of administration brought to a successful conclusion through negotiation and the acceptance of a satisfactory and credible record of payments.

Why were accounts created?

The relatively small number of extant probate accounts is a reflection of how few were created. In the case of Lichfield, for example, an account was drawn up for just 1.4 per cent of all administrations.[9] This begs the question of why they were made in some cases and not others, and whether the under-lying reasons might affect their use for the social history of medicine. A full analysis of the reasons for the creation of probate accounts was carried out in the course of this study.[10] As its conclusions are crucial to the reliability of this book, the major findings are repeated here.

It has long been recognised that some accounts were made at the request of a family member, sometimes a few years after the death.[11] An example of a son requiring his guardian to account for his inheritance, of which there was nothing left (it having been spent on his upbringing over the previous fourteen years), appears in the account of Pleasance Caporne of Brimpton, Berkshire.[12] By comparing pre-1685 and post-1685 accounts, it is possible to assess the proportion of accounts made in this way at the request of the family of the deceased. In Kent this amounted to 25 per cent of all accounts before the act; elsewhere the figure may have been 20 per cent.[13] Thus the great majority were created at the instigation of the courts.

The courts had a number of reasons for requiring an account to be made. A comparison pre- and post-1685 reveals that about 5 per cent of all accounts were required to be made for technical or legal reasons, such as a will being nuncupative, the renunciation of an estate by the widow, or the entering of a *caveat* over the administration of the estate.[14] However, the vast majority were ordered because of debt. It was not necessary for the whole estate to be indebted, only for there to have been a significant level of encumbrance

[8] This quotation comes from *Berkshire probate accounts*, 131, but it is by no means rare.
[9] A. Tarver, 'Understanding probate accounts and their generation in the post-Restoration diocese of Lichfield and Coventry to 1700', in Arkell, Evans and Goose, *When death us do part*, 235.
[10] Mortimer, 'Why were probate accounts made?'
[11] See Tarver, 'Post-Restoration probate accounts', 247–8. She refers to this sort of account as a 'disputed account'.
[12] *Berkshire probate accounts*, 93–4. The account is dated 1601.
[13] Mortimer, 'Why were probate accounts made?', 7.
[14] Ibid. 8.

upon it. Of the 12,579 accounts for East Kent dated 1590–1719 for which a gross estate value (the adjusted value of the probate inventory) is known, 8,299 had debts amounting to more than half of the whole estate or more than £100. While it might possibly be argued that this was representative of the entire community, it would appear far more likely that the accounts were made for indebted estates precisely because of their indebtedness.

Having said this, the proportion of an estate encumbered was not necessarily the direct cause for the court or the family to request an account. The level of expenses is likely to have been a symptom of other, prior concerns. For example, the deceased's ownership of property being contested in a London court may have led to calls for an account, in which case the heavy expenditure was merely a by-product. Similarly, some accounts were rendered much later than the usual one year after the death on account of orphaned beneficiaries who were being cared for at the cost of the estate. Such estates tended to be subject to heavy expenditure over the years of childcare, in clothing, education, washing and schooling the children. Thus the indebtedness of an estate is not necessarily indicative of a court performing a simple financial risk analysis on the strength of a few creditors' claims; it almost certainly represents a longer and more developed process, in which the gross value of the estate and its debts, costs of children's upbringing, servants' wages, rent and status were all taken into consideration. An estate's risk of indebtedness was deemed to arise from a multiplicity of factors, and these factors were what impelled the decision for an account to be made, not just recognised 'debts'. The level of possible expenses was merely the underlying factor, which could only actually be measured after the administration was at an end.

One other important reason underlying the creation of accounts was the division of the estate. Of the 12,579 accounts for East Kent, 4,280 had debts of less than £100 and less than half of the gross value of the estate. Of these 167 related to a nuncupative will, in which case an account was normally called for by the court. Of the remaining 4,113, at least 3,757 were administrations of intestates' estates, where the motivating factor was often the need to distribute the goods of a deceased man or woman fairly among the offspring. A good example is the 1611 account of William Borer; this does not even include funeral expenditure but only the charges of passing the account.[15] The reason for its creation is demonstrated by the detailed allocation of money by the court and the intestacy of the deceased. Overall, 99 per cent of estates which did not have heavy debts were cases in which there was no will or the will was not administered by the appointed executor.[16]

---

15 WSRO, EpI/33/1612/4.
16 I. Mortimer, 'Medical assistance to the dying in provincial southern England, c. 1570–1720', unpubl. PhD diss. Exeter 2004, i. 69. The figure of 4,365 on this page (estates with a balance of more than two-thirds of gross estate value and debts of less than £100) should correctly read 4,465.

Hence it can be said with confidence that, in cases where neither anticipated debts nor legal technicalities were the reason for an account to be made, the determining factors were (1) allocation of estate assets, often at the family's request, and (2) the supervision of administrations of testators' estates where the executor was unable or unwilling to act.

The implications of this are hugely significant for those studying patterns of credit based on probate accounts, but it is unlikely that so financially-skewed a sample will have distorted the representative nature of medical entries. The rich and indebted too fell sick and died, not just the poor. It could be argued that high levels of indebtedness at death were more likely for those who died suddenly, who had not put their affairs in order, and that therefore these accounts are likely to represent an under-recording of payments for medical care. If this is the case, it would mean that this study underestimates the levels of medical and nursing involvement with death. This is less problematic than the possibility that it is prone to overestimates, especially as the prime value of the probate accounts is to reveal changes and trends in the patterns of medical and nursing consumption.

Accessing the accounts

The index to all the probate accounts in England and Wales, created by Peter Spufford in the early 1990s, has greatly facilitated access to the documents. This is partly by way of the published indexes, which appeared in 1999.[17] But far more useful to social historians is the unpublished electronic database. With more than thirty fields for each account, it contains personal details for almost all the deceased people represented, from their name and parish to the name of the executor or the administrator of the estate and his or her relationship to the deceased. It also includes a subject index which, although somewhat erratic, greatly opens up the potential for examining large numbers of documents for a specific type of thematic study.

The database was the starting point for this study. The raw data for eleven counties (including the five main collections listed above) was supplied by the University of Cambridge and reconstituted within a new relational database. The medical and illness indexing for each county were then compared. It was immediately apparent that there are huge contrasts in the data. Only seven of the 656 accounts for Worcestershire are marked on the index as relating to medicine or sickness. At the other extreme, about a quarter of the 13,500 accounts for the diocese of Canterbury – by far the largest collection – include a medical, nursing or illness-related payment. Close examination of the documents and checking against the indexes revealed two important

---

[17] *Index to the probate accounts of England and Wales, A–J*, ed. P. Spufford (British Records Society Ltd, Index Library cxii, 1999).

reasons for the differences (apart from those arising from regional variation in medicalisation). The first is that the researcher who indexed Canterbury was thorough, and indexed all appearances of medical and nursing entries with minimum accuracies of 95 per cent and 90 per cent respectively (with only one identifiable significant slippage from this high standard).[18] The researchers who had dealt with the other collections, on the other hand, did not index accounts containing nursing entries as having medical or illness-related interest. The second reason why the indexes showed very few medical entries in some counties was because of the process of creating the accounts. In some places the court clerk had simply totalled the draft account and omitted the details, thereby obscuring references to medicine and illness.

The consequent disparities in the data reinforced the decision to concentrate upon the largest collections. East Kent (the diocese of Canterbury) not only has more accounts per household than any other area but also the greatest proportion of medical and illness-related index entries.[19] The second largest collection, nearly 6,000 accounts relating to Lincolnshire, could not be investigated for logistic reasons; this made it even more important that all three of the other large collections should be used: Berkshire, Wiltshire and West Sussex (the archdeaconry of Chichester). Fortunately these all have a significant level of medical indexing (although the Wiltshire accounts later proved geographically and methodologically awkward). The 900 accounts for Somerset, with no medical index entries at all, clearly cannot be used in the same way. Oxfordshire and Worcestershire accounts likewise lack medical detail. The series for Hampshire and Cornwall are too partial. The scope for this study was therefore defined as central southern England, as represented by Berkshire, Wiltshire and West Sussex, and the south-east, as represented by East Kent.

Methodological issues

Only a third of the estates examined give the occupation or status of the deceased, including widows described as of 'no occupation'. For the period before 1600 this fraction is just one-eighth. This in itself indicates how much data is absent from these accounts. Just as important is the lack of detail regarding the cause of death. While smallpox and plague are sometimes indicated, this is very often in an incidental way, to explain the high cost of carrying a plague victim to burial, or to explain the high cost of nursing. In some cases there may be indications of such a disease but no firm evidence, such as the account of the widow Jane Johnson, which mentions the airing of her house and the cleaning of her clothes (normally allowable expenses in

---

18 Mortimer, 'Medical assistance', i. 86–7.
19 For numbers see Erickson, 'Using probate accounts', 107.

respect of plague victims).[20] Had this been a family home, and several of the members recorded as buried, an assumption of pestilence would be justified; as this account stands, the question of disease remains unanswered.

These *lacunae* hint at the methodological difficulties of using these accounts for a large-scale survey of changing patterns of behaviour. A similar issue is the question of whether all relevant payments are noted. A number of Kent accounts include the phrase 'unpaid for at his/her death' as a qualifier in an entry, for instance 'paid … for necessaries of meate & drinke the which the deceased Joane Daniell had in the tyme of the sicknes whereof she dyed & unpaid at her death'.[21] It is tempting to ask if only those payments which were unpaid at the time of death are recorded in these accounts. A few examples do hint that this might have been the case. One 1676 entry, 'paid vnto Mr Elvery for phisicke and for a Nurse to attend the accomptant and the deceased in the sicknes of which the said deceased dyed *besides the expences of that sicknes before demanded* 38s', may be a description of a part payment.[22] One 1684 account records a payment to a messenger to go to a physician but no payment to a physician.[23] Similarly a 1690 account has an entry which reads 'for goeing for the doctor to Ashford <for the said deceased>' but no payment to any doctor.[24] While the chance that these messengers did not find the doctor, or he refused to attend, cannot be ruled out they cast doubt on the assumption that all medical payments are recorded.

The situation is further complicated by the possibility that, in some parts of the country, old methods of payment for medical services in instalments (part on administering the medicine, part on completion of the cure) were still used, even as late as the early eighteenth century. While the evidence for such practices is extremely scarce in the probate accounts, part-payments and reduced fees (due to death and thus medical failure) may colour the amounts paid in these accounts.[25] In particular, the 1690 account of Elizabeth Hills suggests an example of a partial payment: 'he paid to Mr Greenstreete *in part of* phisicke by him administred to the said deceased in her sicknes whereof she dyed'.[26]

Problems of partial recording and non-recording of medical services might appear at first as immense methodological shadows, but it seems that only their shadows are large: their actual significance is probably small. The quoted example of a possible part-payment is the only one encountered, and as such it probably does not represent a regular part-payment system but

---

[20] CKS, PRC 2/10/458.
[21] PRC 2/11/203.
[22] PRC 2/37/45.
[23] PRC 2/40/237.
[24] PRC 2/41/176.
[25] I. Mortimer, 'Diocesan licensing and medical practitioners in south-west England, 1660–1780', *Medical History* xlviii (2004), 49–68 at pp. 57, 63.
[26] PRC 2/39/50.

Mr Greenstreet's waiving of some of his fee due to the impoverishment of the estate (which had a balance of just £7). On the question of pre-death medical expenditure going unrecorded in an account, there are many documents which indicate that this was an allowable expense, and that such payments do appear in accounts. One of the clearest examples of a pre-death payment being included is 'for attending on the said deceased att another time in his sicknesse and disbursed for him then'.[27] In addition, it was in the accountant's interests to include payments wherever possible. It should be noted that the two quoted examples of medical services being sought by messengers (and these services not appearing in the account) are the only two found. It is very likely that most medical bills were paid on account throughout this period, as the duration or extent of the involvement of an attending practitioner could not be predicted at the outset of the disease or ailment, and the extent of the medical debt often would have become apparent only after the death. This is also true of nursing services. Given the number of payments for apothecaries' wares, at the end of the seventeenth century in particular, there seems no strong reason to doubt that accountants were normally including such payments whether the money was handed over before or after death.

The most significant methodological problem in using these accounts for medical history is that, across time, the collections are not consistently representative. Since indebtedness affected the numbers of accounts called for, and since the level of indebtedness varied from decade to decade (economically poor decades resulting in a greater level of indebtedness and greater numbers of accounts) differing status levels are reflected in the sample. This means that comparing the totals of medical expenditure in one county in the 1620s with the same county in the 1690s is not straightforward, as the accounts of the latter decade represent a different group of people from the former. For instance in East Kent the average (mean) gross estate value of all the cases for which accounts survive between 1590 and 1619 is £70; for 1690–1719 it is £300. Likewise in Berkshire the mean value of estates increased from £65 to £162 over the same period. These increases cannot be put down to inflation; as Mark Overton has shown in his price indices obtained from probate inventories, prices derived from probate sources in general did not change this dramatically over the seventeenth century.[28] It is evident that increasingly accounts were made for only high-value estates in the latter part of the century, especially after the 1685 act. Any comparison over time has to take into consideration such inconsistencies in the sample.

In many ways the nature of probate accounts and the patterns of their creation and survival define the parameters of any large-scale study based upon

[27] PRC 2/41/178.
[28] M. Overton, 'Prices from probate inventories', in Arkell, Evans and Goose, *When death us do part*, 120–41.

them. In restricting ourselves to large, representative collections there is no option but to study south-east and central southern England. Our sample of 'the dying' is similarly defined by default. It is simply 'those who died' – regardless of whether they knew they were dying or not – a far wider spectrum of people than that usually defined as 'dying' by those who have studied attitudes to death in the seventeenth century.[29] Nevertheless, the scope of the collections chosen – East Kent, West Sussex, Berkshire and Wiltshire, covering nearly 18,000 individuals – is certainly large enough to justify significant generalisations. Moreover, the possibility of studying medicine in the context of a large proportion of the seriously ill – not just those who believed that they were about to die – represents a huge advance on previous studies of death, which have almost entirely excluded medicine. Finally, the theoretical methodological problems affecting this study are slight, if not negligible. The one exception – the significant problem of comparing changing social groups over time – is dealt with in detail in chapter 1.

[29] Mortimer, 'Medical assistance', i. 19–22.

1

The Medicalisation of East Kent

If a sample of all surviving probate accounts were to be taken it would be skewed towards East Kent. Erickson has estimated that roughly one-fifth of all deceased adult male residents of the diocese of Canterbury are represented for the later seventeenth century, and more for the decades prior to the Civil Wars.[1] No other geographical region is comparable. East Kent would also dominate any cross-regional sample because it covers a greater range of dates than any other collection. Even if 10 per cent of the East Kent accounts were to be selected for the years 1570–1719, to make the collection comparable in size with that for West Sussex, it would still heavily outweigh Sussex (and any other county for that matter) at the start and end of the date range.[2] With approximately 13,500 documents, almost all of which fall within the parameters of this study,[3] it is significantly larger than the 10,000 unindexed documents in the Public Records Office relating to the whole province of Canterbury, and more than double the size of the next largest diocesan collection (Lincoln). It is more than four times the size of the collections which relate to the diocese of Salisbury (including its three archdeaconries of Berkshire, Sarum and Wiltshire and its peculiar parishes), which is the next largest geographically related set of documents. Finally, a feature of East Kent's geography is that it has few borders with other administrative areas – the dioceses of Rochester and Chichester being the only two – more than half its border being coastline. Thus Kent represents the best opportunity of examining the financial practices of the dying in a geographical context, and serves as the model upon which this study of provincial medical assistance is built.

Perhaps the easiest way to begin to examine what these documents may tell us about medical services to the dying is to outline what they do not tell us.[4]

---

[1] Erickson, 'Using probate accounts', 105.

[2] Ibid. 107.

[3] A few documents are dated prior to 1570 and some after 1719. The latter have been consulted as far as 1730 for data which may reflect on practitioners whose earlier activities are examined in this book but otherwise these have been ignored. A handful of documents are duplicates relating to a single estate, in which cases only the latest document has been used in an analysis of estates' purchasing of medical services.

[4] The totals given in table 1 do not exactly tally with those in tables 2–5 and 7–8 because they include accounts which have no GEV, balance or occupational descriptor and therefore cannot be placed in the tables according to status.

Table 1
East Kent accounts with medical- and nursing-related entries

Date	Accounts	Medical	Nursing
1570–99	2,340	5%	15%
1600–29	4,808	8%	15%
1630–49	2,319	15%	16%
1660–89	3,418	27%	15%
1690–1719	538	50%	23%
Total	13,423	15%	16%

One superficial message suggested by table 1 is that, as the percentage of paid nursing involvement over the whole period did not change greatly, very little change took place.[5] Similarly, if paid nursing involvement did develop, it only reached the 20 per cent mark in the 1690s, and so was later to expand than medical intervention, which reached the 20 per cent mark in the 1660s. Further investigation shows that these readings of the data are fundamentally unsound and highly misleading. It cannot be taken that over the whole period a static percentage in table 1 represents stasis in the social history of nursing or medical treatment; many different factors may contrive to give the same figure. Similarly, it would be foolish to conclude that only a small proportion of the Kentish population paid for medical services at or near the point of death, or that only a small proportion received nursing treatment, as many of the nursing personnel were members of the household, family and servants, and thus to a large degree outside the scope of the probate account. It might be inferred that the tendency to obtain medical services increased over the period, but even this inference requires qualification, as it will be noticed that only the last four decades show significant proportions of the dying receiving medical assistance, and in these decades the numbers of accounts are low. These are also decades in which the Kent accounts represent estates of far higher value than earlier documents. It is clear that, without more thorough analysis, the trends demonstrated in table 1 are unhelpful.

This unhelpfulness stems from a failure to distinguish specific contexts for changes which might have taken place. All wealth and status groups are pooled, as are both sexes and all geographic regions. Moreover, all medical services are collated; that is to say payments to physicians, apothecaries, surgeons, barber-surgeons, bloodletters, bonesetters, female 'healers' and doctors of physic have all been categorised as 'medical', as well as payments implying the services or involvement of one or more of these groups, such

---

[5] The tables in this book are derived from those in Mortimer, 'Medical assistance', in particular the more detailed versions in vol. ii, appendix 1. Any researcher wanting more specific data than provided here should consult this material.

as payments 'for physic' and 'for medicines' or 'for physical advice'. Thus this column represents any remedial action purchased by or on behalf of the dying patient with reference only to date, nothing else. 'Nursing services' includes any reference to any palliative services, including 'assistance', 'keeping' and 'watching' in the time of the deceased's sickness, as well as nursing (but not wet-nursing or the nursing of children or dependants other than the wife of the deceased where both were simultaneously ill). Again this information has no context apart from date. It is necessary to fragment the totals into their constituent elements, to examine the importance of status, gender and geographic location in the use of services.

Male wealth and status

In breaking up the East Kent data into meaningful groups, it is necessary above all to distinguish those with considerable purchasing power from those with less. There are a number of ways to do this: 'purchasing power' could be defined as wealth, and individuals with high gross or net estate values could be segregated from those with low ones. Alternatively status could be emphasised and 'gentlemen' be singled out from labourers, and their medical experiences at the point of death contrasted. However these approaches are both impractical and open to objection. The wealth of those for whom probate accounts exist varies greatly between counties and over decades, and is not wholly dependent upon the prosperity of society as a whole but on legal and social changes (such as the 1685 act of parliament). Hence relative wealth cannot be used to distinguish the rich from the poor; for example, the poorest 25 per cent of estates in 1660–85 cannot be compared with the poorest 25 per cent in 1686–1710 because the changing reasons for making an account mean that the two samples are very different, the latter being far richer and less representative of society than the former. As for dividing by status, only a third of all these accounts have an occupational or status-related epithet. Nor can a level of wealth be correlated to a high or low status designation; the gross estate values of gentlemen and yeomen varied enormously, as did the wealth of workmen and labourers.[6] Thus the usual means of differentiating between status groups – according to occupation or social rank – is not available.

These problems have forced the development of a unique solution: to optimise the definition of bands of purchasing power by incorporating all

---

6   Of the forty-five labourers in the Kent probate accounts, one had an inventory valued at more than £300, two inventories of more than £100, and twenty-seven inventories of less than £40. Of the 740 designated yeomen, the richest had goods and chattels worth £2,598, the poorest £6 (excluding zero-assessments) and the median £177. Of the 374 gentlemen, the richest had goods and chattels worth £3,528 and the poorest £5, the median being £166.

the evidence available, descriptive as well as quantifiable. The starting point in doing this has been the 'gross estate value' (GEV) of a deceased's estate, largely because amounts of money are easily comparable and this detail exists for more than 90 per cent of all East Kent accounts. However, it is clear from some status designations in the collection that a quantification of wealth by itself can be misleading. It is inappropriate, for example, to compare a gentleman's son and heir, with personal chattels worth £30, resident in his father's house, with a labourer with an identical inventory value. Simple stratification according to inventoried wealth is further complicated by the fact that it was very frequently another individual (not the sick person) who paid, or undertook to pay, the practitioner or nurse. Evidence of this can be seen in the most expense-laden medical accounts, in which almost the whole value of the individual's estate was owing to medical practitioners. In 1635 Thomas Browning's accountant claimed £37 in medical fees although his estate was worth only £22.[7] Hence there is no doubt that the value of the deceased's chattels by itself is a poor indication of ability or willingness to obtain medical help.

The key issue is the power of social networks to provide medical help on behalf of a sick person. This includes the ability of a sick person to be loaned or given money by a wealthy friend or relative. Hence the resource network of a 'gentleman' was normally considerably richer than that of a labourer or husbandman, regardless of their personal inventoried wealth. Conversely, the resource networks of those of lower social status should not be ignored. These may have been less important in obtaining some forms of help and more important in obtaining others. Some nursing services may have been rendered freely more often to those of the same status as the women doing the nursing, for example. Better-off women may have been reluctant to charge their poorer clientele whereas poor women looking after the wealthy were perhaps less likely to waive their fee.

Another reason for not using inventoried wealth in isolation as a measure of purchasing power lies in the relationship between wealth and the capacity to spend. The high levels of indebtedness noted in some of these accounts reveal that it was possible for a man to spend far more than his entire estate was worth. As Craig Muldrew has demonstrated, there was an active credit economy in the seventeenth century in which prices were measured in currency but otherwise there was relatively little relationship between

---

[7] PRC 2/33/12. Other noteworthy instances might include the case of Catherine Symons (PRC 2/36/123), whose stomach cancer drove her from practitioner to practitioner. Before she died she had spent about £32 on medical advice and treatment, although her chattels were worth only £51. Cases of individuals spending more than one-eighth of the value of their chattels on medical care in the seventeenth century are not uncommon. For other examples see PRC 2/35/192, PRC 2/36/3 and PRC 2/40/86.

exchange and hard cash.[8] This has a particular resonance for this study: the merchant who is already £1,000 in debt is hardly likely to put off calling for medical help for the sake of two or three pounds more debt. Indeed, it would be altogether unwise to assume that a certain level of debt means that an estate has reached the limit of its ability to borrow, since indebtedness at death was predicated largely by the timing of the death of the borrower, not by his capacity to borrow. For this reason, regardless of the balance of an account, a high level of indebtedness is evidence of a degree of purchasing power well beyond that implicit in the sum of the inventory.

All such problems are compounded when considering the status of women. Those for whom probate accounts were made – many of them widows – seem to have been more likely than their male counterparts to be resident in another person's house, and thus to have had a lower inventoried wealth, especially before the Civil Wars. The 1617 account of Margaret Charles of Hackington, for example, mentions escutcheons painted 'on mettle' and 20s. given to the poor at her funeral, yet her possessions were worth only £27 4s.[9] It might be supposed that generally the land and income of a woman's husband went to her children, and she was left with little that was her own, even if she did maintain her own house. A check on status in such cases is made harder by the fact that an occupational epithet is rarely present, most women having only a marital condition as a descriptor (although 'gentle-woman' and 'Mrs' may be noted). Thus, although it seems that on average women were less wealthy than men, this does not mean that they were of a lower social status, or had a more limited ability to pay for medical care. If a widow's husband had recently predeceased her, the probate process itself may have reduced her charge significantly, the widow having normally only a third of her husband's estate. This could be sufficient to remove her from one financial group and into another. For example, the charge on the accountant of William Ewell of Herne was £88 19s. 8d., about the average for a tradesman. The balance was £43 5s. 9d. When Ewell's widow died a short while later, her inventory was established at only a pound more than her husband's balance, £44 5s. 9d., the equivalent of the wealthiest labourers. Her account balance was just £21 3s. 8d.[10]

Any assessment of relative purchasing power with regard to medicine must therefore take into consideration the wealth of kinship networks as well as the sex, social status and perceived credit-worthiness of the sick person. To this end the gross estate value has been used as the basic indicator, on the grounds that the average manual labourer did not have £200 of goods in his house, and so a charge of £200 indicates a status above that of the average

[8]   C. Muldrew, 'Hard food for Midas: cash and its social value in early modern England', *Past and Present* clxx (2001), 78–120.
[9]   PRC 2/20/49.
[10] PRC 20/1/195, 207. Another example is that of Henry Burneforde, whose gross estate value was £18 14s. 10d. and whose widow's was £11 9s. 10d.: PRC 2/16/131, 136.

manual labourer. This wealth-based definition is clarified wherever possible, through details such as occupation, title and the ability to borrow (as represented by high levels of indebtedness). While such a methodology results in status bands which only loosely correlate with the status-related titles of 'gentleman', 'skilled worker' and 'labourer' preferred by most social historians, it allows medical expenditure to be examined in more precise social contexts than if all patients were regarded as one undifferentiated mass.

With regard to men, four status groups have been used:

Status A: All males with a gross estate value of £200 or more (including, where this figure is not available, those with a balance of account of £200 or more), or with debts of more than £300 (i.e. balance in excess of £300 in the red, which usually requires debts of considerably more than £300),[11] and those with lower charges and smaller debts described as 'knight' or 'gentleman'.[12]

Status B: All males with a gross estate value of £100–£199 and the two worth less described as 'esquire'.[13]

Status C: All males with a gross estate value of £40–£99 and those worth less described as 'Mr', 'clerk', 'yeoman' or 'doctor'.[14]

Status D: All males with a gross estate value of £0–£39 except those designated as falling into the above categories.

Using these status groups, payments in the probate accounts for medical and nursing services have been quantified (*see* tables 2–5).

Tables 2–5 show an increase in medical and nursing involvement in all status groups across the seventeenth century. Whereas 15–24 per cent of dying patients in 1600 received some form of nursing or medical assistance, by 1700 this had risen to more than 50 per cent for all groups. This was increasingly due to the assistance of a medical practitioner or dispenser of physic; exclusive dependence on helpers, watchers and other nursing assistants declined heavily. It needs to be stressed that this decline was in the exclusive use of nursing services; even in the last thirty-year period about a third of male patients who received some form of medical intervention

---

[11] The reason for pulling this highly indebted section out of the rest is that most individuals with this level of debt who are described in the accounts are described as gentlemen; a number have no epithet however. With this level of debt it is possible that certain of their chattels had been sold before their deaths to pay creditors, or had been passed to family members to avoid them being taken by creditors, and thus their inventories underestimate their moveable wealth.

[12] In the cases of some documents, where neither charge nor balance is available, expenditure in excess of £300 has been used as an indication of Status A.

[13] It is arguable that 'esquire' was usually a status distinction meriting inclusion in the highest category. However, it is also arguable that the word related to the deceased being armigerous, and little more. On account of the lower wealth, it was decided to include these two men in Status B, so as not to exaggerate their status. This was done knowing that, for most purposes, Status B and Status A would be examined together.

[14] Four Wiltshire accounts with no balance or charge details have been added to this category in considering that county in chapter 2.

Table 2
Status A medical and nursing services

Date	Total	Medical or Nursing	Medical only	Nursing only
1570–99	132	26 (20%)	6	13
1600–29	466	102 (22%)	37	37
1630–49	419	116 (28%)	59	24
1660–89	768	274 (36%)	167	32
1690–1719	222	126 (57%)	74	10

Table 3
Status B medical and nursing services

Date	Total	Medical or Nursing	Medical only	Nursing only
1570–99	207	49 (24%)	9	33
1600–29	478	83 (17%)	27	33
1630–49	287	65 (23%)	23	22
1660–89	690	199 (29%)	117	23
1690–1719	104	55 (53%)	39	2

Table 4
Status C medical and nursing services

Date	Total	Medical or Nursing	Medical only	Nursing only
1570–99	518	89 (17%)	15	62
1600–29	1026	185 (18%)	43	105
1630–49	538	138 (26%)	41	64
1660–89	902	275 (30%)	158	47
1690–1719	96	51 (53%)	26	3

Table 5
Status D medical and nursing services

Date	Total	Medical or Nursing	Medical only	Nursing only
1570–99	1,176	175 (15%)	18	131
1600–29	2,148	336 (16%)	61	221
1630–49	740	150 (20%)	49	58
1660–89	739	205 (28%)	94	50
1690–1719	61	31 (51%)	15	4

paid for nursing assistance as well, and this over and above the assistance which would have been rendered in the course of their service by servants and freely by family members. There seems to have been a significant shift in emphasis from paying for purely palliative assistance to employing some degree of medical intervention.

This observation immediately raises the question of when this shift – which may be termed the medicalisation of severe sickness – occurred in East Kent. Given the data, it is to be expected that it took place at different times for different status groups. With regard to Status A and B patients, medical intervention outweighed exclusively palliative care as early as 1600–29. For the remainder, the shift from an exclusively palliative strategy to a predominantly medical one took place after 1630, but even so it was markedly the case by the 1660s–1680s. This counters (with regard to East Kent, at least) Joan Lane's view that 'in the early years of the eighteenth century ... patients were not disposed to seek and pay for advice except in desperate circumstances. By the 1750s, however, patients increasingly came to spend money on more scientific medical attention as part of a higher standard of living'.[15] While it may well be true that patients only sought medical intervention in desperate circumstances, it is clear that long before 1750 the majority of East Kent patients in such situations did so and that medical strategies to cope with life-threatening situations were not restricted to the wealthy.

In order to date the crossover from an exclusive palliative strategy to a predominantly medical one as accurately as possible, figures 1–4 have been drawn up for the four status groups on a decade-by-decade basis. Since all palliative care has been plotted, rather than just nursing exclusive of medicine, the full extent to which medical relief took over from nursing care as the means to alleviate suffering from severe illness in the seventeenth century is demonstrated.

In all status groups nursing care was the most common form of assistance purchased in the late sixteenth century. In the years around 1600 even the best-connected and wealthiest group of patients, Status A individuals, paid for nursing assistance at least as commonly as they paid for medical services. But in all groups the use made of this service tended to stasis or gradual decline until the Civil War. In the 1640s a sharp dip in nursing services is noticeable across all status groups. After the Interregnum an increase in nursing may be noted, first among the accounts of the poorer two categories from the 1670s, and, more gradually, a decade later among the two better-off categories. Only among the less well-off, however, did the increase in the use of nursing services markedly exceed the level of the late sixteenth century. This was nursing care in a slightly different guise: in the earlier period most nursing care for the poorer categories had been conducted without recourse to medical practitioners. In the period 1680–1719 nursing services normally

[15] J. Lane, The social history of medicine, London 2001, 11.

Figure 1
Status A accounts indicating purchase of medical and nursing services

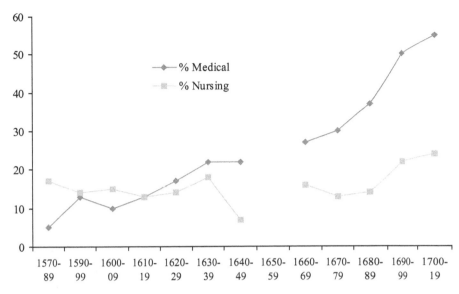

Figure 2
Status B accounts indicating purchase of medical and nursing services

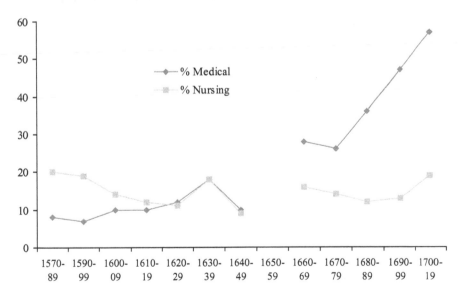

Figure 3
Status C accounts indicating purchase of medical and nursing services

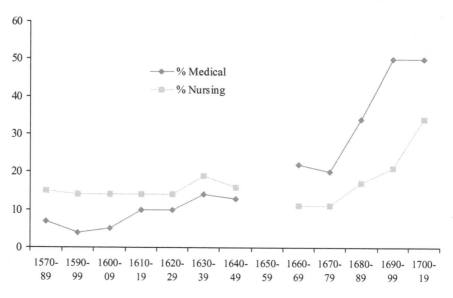

Figure 4
Status D accounts indicating purchase of medical and nursing services

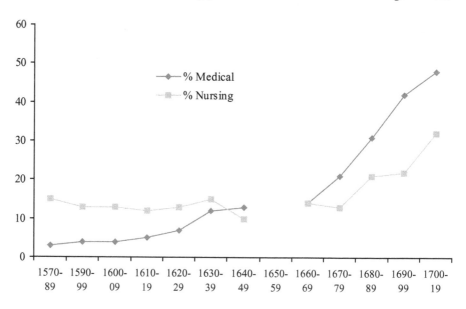

accompanied the services of medical practitioners. For Status C and Status D patients – the group that most frequently used nursing services in isolation in the later decades of this study – only 30 per cent of nursing cases were not accompanied by medical help. For the period 1570–1609 the proportion for these same status groups was 84 per cent.

With regard to medical services, the data suggest a slow growth in use by all classes between 1590 and 1630, the most markedly upward shift being amongst Status A individuals. For this group, the services of apothecaries, surgeons and physicians had become as frequently employed as those of nursing attendants by 1615–25. For other status groups it would appear that the period 1640–60 saw medicine take over as the prime care strategy for seriously ill and dying men, so that by 1675 medical relief was more frequently paid for than nursing care by all. Thereafter the increase in the employment of medical treatment was dramatic. Given that these percentages are *minima* – and must exclude a number of people who died suddenly,[16] or died of predictable weaknesses in old age, tended freely by their families or as part of their duties by household servants, or whose accounts are ambiguous – it can only be concluded that after 1675 the great majority of non-destitute dying people who required medical assistance of some variety not only sought it but obtained it, in some degree at least.

That medical care was the predominant form of assistance purchased by all status groups by 1675 does not automatically imply that medical services were as easily available to the poor as they were to the wealthy. Indeed, it does not imply that the medical services which the less well-off obtained were even comparable with those purchased by the wealthy. The only aspect which is directly comparable is the adoption of a medical strategy (i.e. a course of action which involved paying a medical practitioner) as opposed to a purely palliative one. While there seems to have been very little difference in the propensity of the separate groups to obtain nursing care before the 1680s, the stratification of wealth highlights a consistently greater propensity among the better-off to obtain medical care.

Status groups C and D closely follow A and B in the purchase of medical and nursing care. Although there is a clear line of demarcation in the purchasing of medical help, the proportion of the lower status groups obtaining medical services was normally above two-thirds of the proportion of the higher status groups. To be precise, in East Kent over the period 1570–1689 the propensity of Status C and D patients to obtain medical care compared to Status A and B was 1:1.67. Yet there is a marked difference between the wealth of these groups. At no point in the period under study does the mean GEV of groups C and D reach even a fifth of that of status groups A and B. Wealth and status were of relatively little consequence in deciding whether to obtain nursing help and palliative assistance, and of

---

16 This group is estimated at 6% in chapter 5.

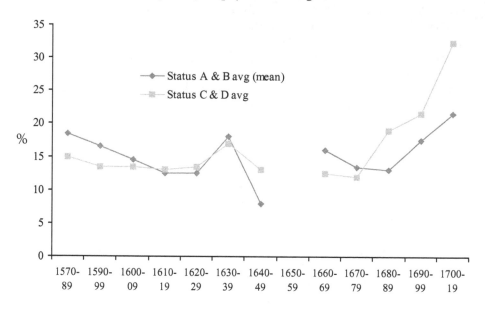

Figure 5
Propensity to pay for nursing services

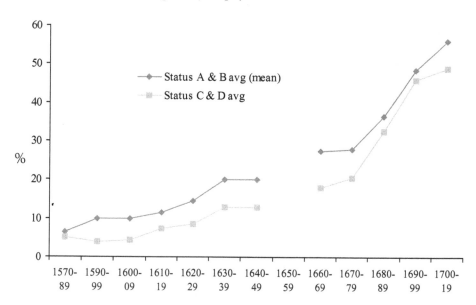

Figure 6
Propensity to pay for medical services

minor significance in considering whether to pursue a medical strategy to deal with a serious medical condition. They played an important part in deciding the type of medical help sought, but not whether medical intervention was desirable in principle.

That said, it remains a moot point whether the poor could afford medical help. To what extent does a band of several thousand men with chattels worth less than £40 represent the poor? If they were so poor, why was an account called for by the courts? Those who had few or no chattels were unlikely to have very heavy debts and nor did they have estates to be divided among their offspring. The best that can be done to test the findings for the 'poor' is to single out the poorest section of the poorest group, those with gross estate values of between £1 and £10. Unfortunately changes post-1630 cannot be traced, as these estates are only significantly represented for the years 1570–1630, but a comparison of their propensity to pay for medical and nursing services by comparison with the others in the lowest financial bracket is possible. Table 6 indicates that the proportion of accounts which include a payment for medical or nursing care is comparable with Status D patients as a whole except for the fact that very few paid for a medical strategy. Of the one in six poor who did pay for some help in 1570–1629, just 7 per cent paid for medicine. Of the other Status D patients – those with £10-£39 of chattels – this figure was 17 per cent.

Table 6
East Kent accounts for deceased males with estates less than £10

Date	Total	Medical or Nursing	Medical only	Nursing only
1570–99	239	38 (16%)	3	30
1600–29	223	36 (16%)	2	30

In conclusion, the seventeenth century saw a number of developments in the pattern of medical and nursing consumption amongst males in East Kent. Four general points may be established. First, there was a significant shift in the strategies used to deal with extreme medical situations, from initial reliance upon purely palliative care towards a widespread reliance upon a medical strategy (often in conjunction with nursing care). This shift took place over the course of the period 1610–60. Second, this resulted in a marked increase in the absolute level of medical care purchased over the entire period, accelerating most for the lower status groups in the decades 1670–89. Third, there is a slight but consistent discrepancy in the propensity to adopt a medical strategy between the various status groups, which might reflect the ability to obtain such assistance but which, if so, is less significant than has normally hitherto been presumed. And fourth, there is evidence of a revival in the importance of paid palliative assistance, especially to the less well-off, towards the end of the seventeenth century.

Gender

To run a direct comparison between men and women of similar status groups is slightly misleading. Widows in particular tend to be placed in a lower financial bracket than the men to whom they had been married.[17] This being an inconsistent discrepancy, and the original delineations of wealth in respect of status being arbitrary, there is no way systematically to correlate the use of medical and nursing strategies adopted by men and women in relation to status. However, it is possible to run similar experiments with the data to see what medical services were purchased by women of varying status levels and to compare the trends with those observed with regard to men.

In tables 7 and 8, Status R has been assigned to those women (almost always widows and spinsters) who, on the financial or social grounds already outlined, would have qualified for status group A or B if they had been male.[18] This is the distinct minority of females for whom accounts were made (18 per cent). The majority is made up by women in Status S, defined by the same criteria as define groups C and D.

Table 7
Status R medical and nursing services (females)

Date	Total	Medical or Nursing	Medical only	Nursing only
1570–99	26	7 (27%)	1	5
1600–29	80	31 (39%)	6	13
1630–49	66	29 (44%)	8	11
1660–89	119	49 (41%)	24	7
1690–1719	30	16 (53%)	7	3

Table 8
Status S medical and nursing services (females)

Date	Total	Medical or Nursing	Medical only	Nursing only
1570–99	253	62 (25%)	6	47
1600–29	580	168 (29%)	24	113
1630–49	263	78 (30%)	18	43
1660–89	300	101 (34%)	37	28
1690–1719	24	12 (50%)	4	3

[17] For example, compare PRC 2/41/155 and PRC 2/41/154. The latter is the husband, whose chattels were valued at £298, and the former was his wife, whose chattels were estimated to be worth £83.

[18] It is usually said that married women could not make a will. However, in theory they could if they had their husband's permission. No unambiguous example has been identified among these accounts of a married woman's estate being formally executed by her husband. One possibility is that of the 'widow' Elizabeth Drust, formerly Sheafe, whose 'relict', Robert Drust, administered her estate in 1623: PRC 2/24/87. Another possible case is that of Dorothie Ungleye, 'widow', whose estate was administered by her 'relict' John Alcocke in 1609: PRC 2/14/460.

Both female status groups show trends similar to their male counterparts. There is a marked increase in the propensity to pay for medical and nursing services over the whole period. There is a clear decrease in the proportion of female patients who paid only for palliative care commensurate with a marked increase in the proportion of those adopting a medical strategy. In addition, just as the wealth and status of deceased males made a consistent but surprisingly slight difference in the propensity to pay for medical help, so too Status R women were only slightly more likely to pay for medical services than Status S. This is interesting considering the large difference in estate values between Status R (with a mean GEV of £257) and Status S (£30). Conversely it may be noted that the less well-off paid for nursing assistance more regularly throughout the period, possibly on account of a restricted ability to rely on domestic servants and resident kin.

Given that most of the trends noted for deceased males are also observable for deceased females, it is justifiable to question whether there are any significant differences in the extent to which the sexes adopted medical and nursing strategies. A limited degree of comparison is possible by comparing status groups A and B with status group R. The two groups vary greatly in the proportions of the whole sample which they represent at each time, and they vary widely in the bands of wealth they cover as well as the relative status levels of each sex, but they may be compared on the grounds that they represent the wealthiest, the most economically versatile and the most socially distinguished elements of the community.

Figure 7 indicates that the level of nursing care obtained by better-off women compares with that obtained by better-off men. However, although medical strategies were more commonly sought than palliative assistance on behalf of dying males from about the mid 1610s; for single females this was not the case before the Interregnum. This was not due to a greater reluctance to obtain medical care (usually administered by men) on the part of the females: it was due to a far higher rate of purchase of palliative care. Roughly two-thirds of all nursing care shown here was to help dying women.[19] It seems safe to say that the nursing services available to the better-off were not only dominated by women but also largely for the benefit of women. Men in status groups A and B, we might presume, depended more on their wives, servants and resident kinfolk than paid nursing assistance.

The differences between the sexes among the middling to poorer sort were minimal with regard to medical expenditure. Again, the difference between the sexes in the use of paid assistance lay in nursing: single women more frequently made use of nursing services than men. Furthermore, the

[19] The proportions of nursing care obtained for females from the total for status groups A and B (males) and R (females) are as follows: 1570–99 61%; 1600–29 69%; 1630–[49] 70%; 1660–89 60%; 1690–1719 57%; mean: 63.4%. These figures are based on the percentages of females obtaining nursing services in relation to percentages of males and females obtaining them.

Figure 7
Propensity to pay for medical and nursing services: higher status groups

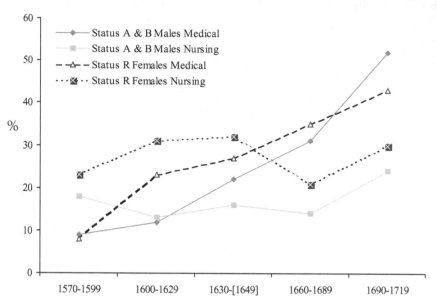

Legend:
- Status A & B Males Medical
- Status A & B Males Nursing
- Status R Females Medical
- Status R Females Nursing

Figure 8
Propensity to pay for medical and nursing services: lower status groups

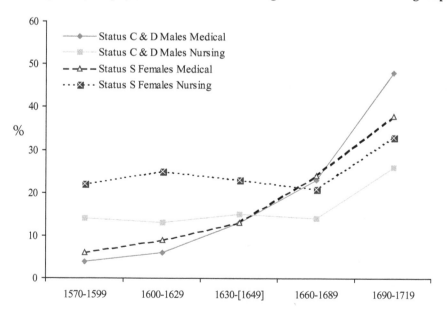

Legend:
- Status C & D Males Medical
- Status C & D Males Nursing
- Status S Females Medical
- Status S Females Nursing

difference is almost the same as it is for status groups A and B. The proportion of nursing care expended on Status S women is only 0.5–1 per cent lower than for Status R women.[20] Women were almost twice as likely to be consumers of nursing care as men before 1690.

The higher proportion of women who sought nursing assistance does not necessarily imply that women more frequently saw nursing and non-occupational medicine as the preferred strategy for coping with health issues or old age. The women for whom probate accounts were made were single, and thus, unlike their married male counterparts, were not able to rely on the care of a spouse. As shown in table 56 (*see* chapter 5), accounts drawn up by a female next of kin of deceased males were roughly half as likely to incorporate nursing services as those drawn up by male executors and administrators. Women tending the sick and dying were not always wives, of course; daughters and sisters might also play a palliative role, relieving a household of the need to pay for nursing care (whether it be that of a dying man or woman). However, as 92 per cent of the females administering a man's estate were widows, it is safe to say that the key difference underlying male and female nursing was the nursing role of wives.

In conclusion, dying men and women of roughly comparable status sought medical remedies to serious health threats with a comparable readiness over the course of the seventeenth century. The important difference between their approaches to assistance lay in the purchase of nursing services, i.e. non-occupational medical help and general household 'help in the time of the sickness'. Women were twice as likely to obtain nursing care as men. If married women (unrepresented in these accounts), were as likely to obtain nursing care as single women, it could be said that 65 per cent of all paid nursing care was obtained on behalf of females in the period 1570–1690.

Geography: medical services

There are a number of possible approaches to the geography of medical services. The most obvious and arguably the most important line of enquiry in the wake of Margaret Pelling's findings is the question of whether and to what extent towns acted as medical centres, and whether they dominated the distribution of medical services to the detriment of rural areas.[21] Thus the first subject to address is the basic issue of what is meant by 'town' in East Kent in the early modern period.

---

[20] The proportions of Status S females of all three less well-off social groups purchasing nursing services are 1570–99 61%; 1600–29 66%; 1630–49 61%; 1660–89 70%; 1690–1719 56%; mean: 62.8%.

[21] Pelling and Webster, 'Medical practitioners', 165–236, especially with reference to the work on population: practitioner ratios in the conclusion at pp. 232–6. See also the refinement of the Norwich statistics in Pelling, 'Tradition and diversity', 159–71.

As Jacqueline Bower has pointed out, there was confusion even at the time as to what constituted a town.[22] Leland (writing in the 1540s), Lambarde (1570s) and Norden (1620s) all give differing lists of towns for the county. Moreover, even those which they all included were not necessarily 'towns' for the purposes of this study, in that they did not have a sufficiently diverse economic base to act as a centre for medical services. Some places, Bower points out, were indisputably towns, such as Canterbury, Dover and Maidstone. But there were about twenty other settlements in East Kent with a market of some description, some with populations under 500, for example Appledore and Sutton Valence. In these places the existence of a market – an agricultural economic marker – cannot be considered a satisfactory measure of the availability of a range of medical services. John Norden's list of towns in 1625, for example, includes Lenham – with which only five medical practitioners can be associated – and excludes Tenterden, with seventeen.[23] Thus any list of market towns or settlements, whether based on a contemporary authority or in retrospect, is bound to be a somewhat arbitrary starting point from which to examine the role of urban settlements in providing medical services.

In view of this problem, and since this study concentrates upon a very specific and distinct aspect of town life, a more appropriate definition has been adopted. This is to assess 'medical towns' by the number of practitioners resident in each place over the period 1570–1720. The logic behind this may clearly be seen by the modern parallel: not all modern towns have a hospital, although towns are crucially important today in the provision of medical care to the dying. 'Medical towns' are therefore defined as any settlement with nine or more known practitioners: no parish has seven or eight, and only two market towns have six.[24] The result is a list of fifteen 'medical towns': Ashford, Canterbury, Cranbrook, Deal, Dover, Elham, Faversham, Hythe, Maidstone, Milton, New Romney, Sandwich, Sittingbourne, Tenterden and Wye. This list includes all but four of Lambarde's active market towns (Appledore, 6 practitioners; Lenham, 5; Smarden, 6; and Sutton Valence, 2). Of the fifteen, Milton and Sittingbourne are closely situated, less than a mile apart, and may be regarded as one. Lydd (6 practitioners) and New Romney are similarly closely located (three miles apart, Lydd being an appurtenance of the liberty of Romney), with a combined practitioner contingent of fifteen over the period. Of the places selected which do not appear in Lambarde's list – Tenterden, Sittingbourne and Deal – the justification for regarding these as medical towns in the same way as

---

[22] J. Bower, 'Kent towns, 1540–1640', in M. Zell (ed.), *Early modern Kent, 1540–1640*, Woodbridge 2000, 141–76.

[23] I. Mortimer, 'A directory of medical personnel qualified and practising in the diocese of Canterbury, c. 1560–1730', *Archaeologia Cantiana* cxxvi (2006), 135–69. This is based on Mortimer, 'Medical assistance', ii, appendix 2.

[24] Idem, 'Medical assistance', i. 113–14.

market places lies in the perceived danger of ignoring them. For example, to discount Tenterden with its seventeen practitioners as a centre and to regard it merely as being a 'rural' parish seven miles from the nearest 'town', Cranbrook, with its sixteen practitioners, is to miss the point of examining towns as medical foci. In addition it should be noted that all three of these places had other claims to town status. Sittingbourne was incorporated in the reign of Elizabeth, and so might be said to have been growing into town status at the time Lambarde was writing; it is also adjacent to Milton and so may be said to have had a local market. Tenterden was granted a new charter by Elizabeth in 1599–1600.[25] Both Sittingbourne and Tenterden had been described as towns by Leland in the Tudor period, so their roots as local centres were long-established. Finally Deal, one of the Cinque Ports (as a dependency of Sandwich), was incorporated by charter towards the end of the period under study, in 1698–9.[26] Thus all the places selected may be said to have been towns of some sort by 1700.

Using these fifteen towns as medical foci, and the areas around them as medical hinterlands, we may turn to the map. No point in East Kent is more than 8.5 miles from one of these towns. Apart from a small section on the coast in the parishes of Chislet and St Nicholas at Wade, and a patch on the tip of the Isle of Thanet, the only area which is more than seven miles from a 'medical town' is a four-square-mile area along the border of the parishes of Lenham and Boughton Malherbe. Lenham was a market town with five medical practitioners over the period, and so has some justification to be regarded as a minor medical centre in its own right. Thanet too had more practitioners than most rural places.

The important question is whether this apparently even spread of medical towns and practitioners was sufficient to allow medical services to be obtained by rural communities as easily as urban ones. In addition, was the residence of a practitioner in a locality sufficient guarantee that he could be found and persuaded to serve all the nearby communities?

In order to examine this subject, each parish in the diocese of Canterbury has been assigned to the catchment area of its nearest 'medical town' up to a distance of six miles.[27] The areas beyond this distance – the area around Lenham and parts of Thanet and Sheppey – have been associated with Lenham, Sandwich and Milton respectively. Thus Birchington appears associated with Sandwich, at a distance of seven miles. Sheppey parishes have been associated with Milton rather than Faversham, due to the crossing point over the Swale being nearer Milton. Areas equidistant from two

25 Kellys directory of Kent, London 1939, 664.
26 Ibid. 226.
27 Measurements have, for the most part, been taken from Bartholomews gazetteer, 9th edn, London 1943, repr. 1966. In certain instances, where this gives a distance to a town other than the nearest medical one, the measurement has been calculated 'as the crow flies' (like Bartholomews) from the parish church.

'medical towns' have been associated with the more significant one, based on the number of practitioners associated with it. Nonington, whose centre is unique in being roughly equidistant – between 6.5 and 7 miles – from five 'medical towns' (Canterbury, Sandwich, Deal, Dover and Elham) has been placed in the catchment area of Canterbury, at a distance of seven miles. Tables 9 and 10 show the levels of medical services for males in relation to all 'medical towns', including Rye in Sussex (four miles from Wittersham) and Lenham in respect of those parishes in its vicinity which are more than six miles from any other 'medical town'.

Table 9
Medical payments in relation to distance fromm medical towns,
Status A & B males

Date	<1 mile %	1–3 miles %	>3 miles %
1570–99	9	6	9
1600–29	18	8	10
1630–49	25	19	16
1660–89	34	37	28
1690–1719	49	53	53

Table 10
Medical payments in relation to distance from medical towns,
Status C & D males

Date	<1 mile %	1–3 miles %	>3 miles %
1570–99	6	2	4
1600–29	10	6	4
1630–49	17	13	10
1660–89	26	26	20
1690–1719	52	52	43

It appears that, prior to the Interregnum, people generally experienced a higher level of medical help if they were resident in or close to 'medical towns' as opposed to living in the hinterland (1–3 miles) or in rural areas (more than 3 miles). This was a period when expenditure on medical services was becoming more common: it might thus be postulated that in these early years of expansion the towns remained important channels of medical business, perhaps catalytic in changing popular attitudes to medicine as well as facilitating its supply. Patients of all status groups in rural areas were able to obtain medicine, although it may well have been harder for them to do so than in towns, especially if they were of low status. By 1690 there was no significant 'medical disadvantage' to those facing severe illness in a town hinterland, and only a slight medical disadvantage in being more than 3 miles from a medical town. Lower levels of medical help for Status C and D than Status A and B are to be noted across all areas, but rarely was the level of rural and hinterland medical intervention less than 50 per cent of that in the medical towns. Even if Status D individuals are isolated, prior to the 1650s, rural dwellers were about half to two-thirds as likely to obtain medical help as their counterparts in a medical town.[28] After that date Status D men in urban hinterlands were just as likely to obtain medical help as town-dwellers, and those in more remote areas were only slightly disadvantaged by their location.

On the strength of the evidence for East Kent, Evenden-Nagy's claim that most of England was medically remote in the seventeenth century may be disregarded.[29] It is possible that East Kent was medically far advanced on other areas of the country, such as the rural north-west of England, but such was the level of medical practitioner availability in East Kent that great caution should be exercised before assuming that any region was completely isolated from medical help. Having said this, the model outlined above is only a general one: it does not allow the assertion that every part of the diocese had access to practitioners. The remotest areas from the medical towns have been lumped together with areas just three miles from such a settlement. Also, in comparing the propensity of rural parishioners to obtain medical help with denizens of 'medical towns' there is an assumption that the medical towns were all equally well-serviced, which they were not. Furthermore, some of the more 'remote' areas (besides Lenham) had a claim themselves to be considered towns: Smarden and Appledore are obvious examples. What is required in order to contextualise these workings is an examination of the most and least 'remote' parts of the diocese, in order to determine whether it is possible to say that any part was indeed medically remote and, if so, to what degree in comparison to the medically best-provisioned towns.

Table 11 is a comparison of medical services purchased in Canterbury, plus the next rank of 'medical towns' – Maidstone, Dover and Sandwich – and the four parishes of the Isle of Thanet, which may be considered one of the most remote parts of the diocese. Prior to the Interregnum, fatal illness was consistently less medicalised in Thanet than in both Canterbury and the second tier of medical towns, despite the greater average wealth of those dying in Thanet for whom accounts were made.[30] Around 1660–70 the situation changed. This is borne out by data relating to the local supply as well as consumption of physic and medical expertise: only three of the ten practitioners who may be associated with the four Thanet parishes were

---

28 Mortimer, 'Medical assistance', ii. 29.
29 D. Nagy, *Popular medicine in seventeenth century England*, Bowling Green 1988, 18.
30 Mortimer, 'Medical assistance', ii. 30.

Table 11
Medical care within, or within one mile of, the principal medical towns compared with parishes in the Isle of Thanet

Date	Canterbury %	Maidstone, Sandwich, Dover %	Isle of Thanet %
1570–99	13	7	4
1600–29	18	14	5
1630–49	25	24	11
1660–89	26	34	27
1690–1719	37	45	62

Note: Table based on data from all status groups, males and females.

licensed before 1650; the other seven (six diocesan licentiates and one arch-diocesan) were all licensed after 1660. So too was the one practitioner who may be associated with the neighbouring parish of St Nicholas at Wade. This goes some way towards explaining why Thanet, one of the most remote parts of the county, was able to provide its dying people with medical care as frequently as the four principal 'medical towns' after the Interregnum. The introduction of local medical practitioners in the latter part of the century greatly facilitated access to medical care in Thanet, and moreover, having relatively few people to serve and shorter distances to travel, it appears that these practitioners were able to provide a level of coverage beyond that of even the best-provisioned medical towns, which seem to have served their hinterlands as much as their citizens or townsmen.

Was Thanet the only part of East Kent that may be seen in this light: medically remote before the Interregnum and better-served than the towns after 1660? It is difficult to distinguish other suitable sample areas, but two demand testing. The first of these is the Isle of Sheppey. Here there were seven parishes – Eastchurch, Elmley, Harty, Leysdown, Minster in Sheppey, Queenborough and Warden – separated from the north of the county by the Swale and reached by a ferry between Iwade and Minster in Sheppey. For this reason, although much of the island is within six miles of Faversham, Milton is the nearest 'medical town', six miles or less from approximately half the island. The second area which may be singled out is Romney Marsh, at the opposite side of the county, a stretch of low-lying land usually said to encompass all the land between Hythe and Rye but which is technically much smaller, only 24,000 acres.[31] The interesting factor here is not so much

---

[31] S. Lewis, *Topographical dictionary of England*, 7th edn, London 1849.

Table 12
Medical care in parishes in the Isle of Sheppey and Romney Marsh

Date	Isle of Sheppey %	Romney Marsh %
1570–99	7	2
1600–29	9	8
1630–49	14	12
1660–89	33	30
1690–1719	[29]	[80]

Note: Table based on data from all status groups, males and females. 1690–1719 based on small sample size: 4/14 (Sheppey) and 8/10 (Romney).

the remoteness of the place – it lies around New Romney, a minor medical town – but the high level of mortality associated with it by Mary Dobson in her *Contours of death*. For the purposes of this study, the parishes included in the Romney Marsh sample include Broomhill (no accounts), Hope All Saints, Ivychurch, Lydd, Midley, New Romney, Old Romney and St Mary in the Marsh.

Leaving aside the unreliably small sample for the last period, the figures for these remote areas seem marginally to exceed those for Thanet. All show a very similar increase in the level of medical services employed, to the extent that they all compare with the largest 'medical towns' by 1660–89. The development in Romney Marsh – a low-lying area known for its high mortality, much of it due to malaria – is particularly remarkable. The most likely explanation for its initial very low level of medical help is that, prior to 1600, there were few or no practitioners resident in the area. In ascertaining this we are heavily dependent on licensing records, and these by no means cover all practitioners (though they cover more in East Kent than elsewhere), but, taken together with the occupational descriptors in marriage licences, records of town freedoms and records of degrees awarded, as well as practitioners mentioned in the accounts themselves, they may serve as an indicator of numbers of practitioners in a region. Robert Pell, active from 1608 to 1629, may have begun his career in Lydd a little earlier than 1608, and Christopher Waters, licensed in 1600, may have practised in New Romney before his licence was granted, but otherwise the nearest identified practitioner was Thomas Thornell in Appledore (licensed 1592). Before that date the nearest places where practitioners could certainly be found were Hythe and Ashford, approximately ten and twelve miles respectively from Lydd. In terms of being medically remote, Romney Marsh seems to have been very much a medical backwater until 1600.

With regard to Sheppey, a total of eight practitioners can be connected

33

with the area during the whole period (to 1720).[32] Two of these were in Queenborough (one licensed 1705; another, Thomas Waferer, began his career in Sittingbourne in or before 1623 and moved to Queenborough before 1639), three in Minster (two licensed in 1635 and 1695, and another active in 1664), one in Eastchurch (licensed 1692) and two in Warden (licensed in 1662 and 1669). But although this suggests that the Isle of Sheppey was less well-serviced than Romney Marsh, most of it lies within six miles of Milton and Sittingbourne, where at least one licensed practitioner (Peter Spurway) was resident in the sixteenth century, and possibly more (for example John Freeman, licensed there in 1600). Three other practitioners were active in Milton between 1600 and 1650, and five more in Sittingbourne.

This offers a simple model of the geographical factors affecting the use of medical services in the diocese. From this may be drawn some provisional conclusions. Most important, some rural areas in the south-east were still medically remote in the sixteenth century, fewer were in the early seventeenth century but probably none were remote after the Restoration. However, the simplicity of the model masks the fact that it depends on an unverified assumption. Drawing up a list of 'medical towns' and suggesting 'catchment areas' – a logical *modus operandi* on the face of it – does not take into consideration the qualitative aspects of medical service and the logistics of fatal illness and injury. Mere residential proximity to a medical town does not necessarily imply that medical help was always obtained from that particular town. People who were injured or fell ill away from home would frequently have sought help elsewhere. A local practitioner might have been unable or unwilling to act in some circumstances. Certain individuals summoned 'their' physician to them from wherever he happened to be, regardless of the nearest medical town or his distance from their own residence (*see* chapter 3). Some practitioners had reputations which preceded them, so that even inhabitants of, say Ashford, might have sought help from specialists in Canterbury or Sandwich rather than their own home town. The bottom line is that such a model cannot be complete if the assumption that there was a strong (if not direct) relationship between proximity to medical services and their consumption cannot be verified.

Such verification is not easy. Any corrective checks on the existing body of data would naturally be based on a similar series of arbitrary decisions about what constitutes a medical town and its hinterland and, ultimately, would be subject to the same assumption as outlined above (or its antithesis). To try to identify the home town of each practitioner named by using licensing and other records would similarly result in a methodological weakness, as it is not always possible to say that a practitioner of one name may certainly be identified with one of the same name in another place, and

---

[32] Mortimer, 'Directory'. This figure might be nine if one counts Thomas Wignall, who might have resided in Minster in Thanet or Minster in Sheppey.

Table 13
Employment of practitioners from the nearest town

Date	< 1 mile	1–3 miles	>3 miles
1570–99	4/6	0/1	5/12
1600–29	84/99	14/24	21/48
1630–49	69/85	18/37	23/42
1660–89	31/51	25/31	34/71
1690–1719	4/4	2/4	4/9
1570–1719	78%	61%	48%

Note: Columns refer to the number of named practitioners described as from the nearest medical town in relation to the total number of practitioners whose place of residence is given. Table based on male and female patients, all status groups.

in making such connections a geographical bias is inevitably introduced. However, by concentrating only on those accounts which themselves specify the place of residence of the medical practitioner employed, an estimate of the relevance of the nearest 'medical town' to patients employing medical practitioners may be obtained.[33]

Table 13 suggests that there is a strong (but by no means exclusive) relationship between close proximity to a medical town and its role as the supplier of medical services locally. About four-fifths of those resident in those towns who sought medical help did so exclusively locally. Given that some people died or fell ill away from home, and a few no doubt sought particular practitioners from further afield, this may be considered a very high proportion, and it might therefore be concluded that the decision to examine these towns as medical *foci* was a good one. But the implications of the figures for the inhabitants of more distant parishes are perhaps even more telling. The assumed relationship between proximity to and supply of medical services becomes less acceptable the further the patient lived from the town. For those in more distant hinterlands – in excess of three miles – the nearest town was still important for the supply of medical help but only to the extent that it was used as a medical centre as often as not (48 per cent of cases). This varied according to the size of the town's medical strength.

While the general analysis suggested that the list of 'medical towns' was justified, it seems clear from table 14 that some places – notably Cranbrook Deal, New Romney and Wye – did not act as a medical *foci* in the same way as, say, Dover, Maidstone and Canterbury. Not surprisingly, the importance of a town to its locality seems to have been heavily dependent on the number of practitioners associated with it. Those with few practitioners were no

---

[33] Very close settlements have been regarded as the same medical town in table 13. This includes Milton and Sittingbourne, Lydd and New Romney, and Ospringe and Faversham.

Table 14
Medical towns in relation to demand for practitioners
based within that town

Town	Practitioners assoc. with town	Named <1 mile	Named 1–6 miles	Total, 0–6 miles
Canterbury	>100	62/65	17/22	79/87
Maidstone	44	10/11	20/25	30/36
Sandwich	33	22/24	7/14	29/36
Dover	40	20/24	5/8	25/32
Faversham	26	32/40	13/23	45/63
Ashford	22	13/17	18/25	31/42
Tenterden	17	9/13	7/16	16/29
Milton and Sittingbourne	36	9/16	16/32	25/48
Hythe	12	5/7	14/30	19/37
Elham	11	3/4	2/6	5/10
Deal	16	1/4	3/6	4/10
Cranbrook	16	3/6	3/11	6/17
New Romney	9	1/6	4/17	5/23
Wye	10	0/6	0/2	0/8
(Lenham)	(5)	1/2	1/6	2/8
(Rye, Sussex)	–	–	2/2	2/2

Note: The last three columns refer to the number of named practitioners described as from the town in relation to the total number of practitioners whose place of residence is given. Table based on male and female patients, all status groups.

different from rural parishes, serving perhaps a small locality with regularity but not consistently meeting all its needs. The six largest medical towns served both their denizens and their hinterlands with impressive consistency. Their hinterlands also seem to have been much broader, overlapping with the hinterlands of smaller towns. Indeed, if ranges of 8.5 mile radii are drawn around each of these six towns it is apparent that almost the whole diocese is covered, with the exceptions of the south fringe, which is served at closer quarters by Cranbrook, Tenterden, New Romney and Hythe. The implication is that, in most of the diocese, living only one mile or two from a minor medical town was medically less important in the event of serious illness than being five miles from a major one. For instance, the inhabitants of Acrise were only a mile from Elham but were five miles from Hythe and eight from Dover: in the face of serious ailments these latter places served as medical centres more frequently than Elham itself.

This finding is of much more than regional importance. Previously understanding of levels of medical coverage in the early modern period has relied heavily on Margaret Pelling's work on sixteenth-century practitioners.[34] In each case studied, London, Norwich and smaller towns such as King's Lynn, it was urban practitioner/population ratios which were examined. Although the ratios of 1:400 in London and 1:200 in Norwich may be technically correct, they do not reflect that, for these cities (the largest two in the country), the population they would have served was much greater than the urban population in their immediate vicinity. Consider, for example, early seventeenth-century Canterbury. There were more than 6,000 – perhaps 7,000 – people living in the city.[35] Applying the methodology of 'Medical practitioners', in the thirty years between 1610 and 1639 there were at least forty-four resident medical practitioners who were licensed by a bishop or archbishop, held a medical degree, received the freedom of the city, or first practised medicine, pharmacy or surgery as noted in the probate accounts. The actual number of practitioners was undoubtedly higher than this, as shown from the probate records of other practitioners not included in that number. However, restricting calculation to what is certain, at least forty-four medical men (all the recorded occupational practitioners were men) were serving a population of up to 7,000. This equates to a practitioner: population ratio of 1:159. However, based on the findings above it is likely that about 77 per cent of the rural hinterland, up to 6 miles from the city, also depended, when in danger of death, on these practitioners. There are thirty-five parishes outside the city whose churches lie within six miles.[36] If these parishes have just the average parish population of 250, then the population within the six-mile hinterland was about 8,750, and 77 per cent of this figure – 6,737 – suggests that the forty-four Canterbury practitioners were catering to as many people within six miles of Canterbury as within the walls.[37] The

34 Pelling and Webster, 'Medical practitioners'; Pelling, 'Tradition and diversity'.
35 Bower, 'Kent towns, 1540–1640', 145.
36 This includes the extra-parochial district of Dunkirk. The other parishes included as outside Canterbury but whose churches are within six miles as the crow flies are Adisham, Bekesbourne, Bishopsbourne, Blean, Boughton under Blean, Bridge, Chartham, Chilham, Chislet, Fordwich, Hackington, Harbledown, Herne, Hoath, Ickham, Kingston, Littlebourne, Lower Hardres, Milton, Nackington, Patrixbourne, Petham, Seasalter, Selling, Stodmarsh, Sturry, Swalecliffe, Thanington, Upper Hardres, Waltham, Westbere, Whitstable, Wickhambreaux and Wingham. *The Compton Census of 1676: a critical edition*, ed. A. Whiteham (British Academy, Records of Social and Economic History x, 1986), gives the adult population of these parishes, not including Blean or Dunkirk, as 4,538. Including children this almost certainly relates to a population in the region well in excess of 7,000, as many parishes have rounded figures of 'about 200' and some seem to have excluded women: ibid. 19–33.
37 Average parish population is estimated by taking the probable population of the diocese of 75,600 and dividing it by 295 parishes. In fact, parishes in the Canterbury hinterland are likely to have been more populous than this. Thus, although 75,600 might be as much as a 10% overestimate of the population of the diocese in 1610–40 (based on Chalklin's estimates for the county in 1676), this figure has not been adjusted downwards

revised practitioner: population ratio for the area as a whole would thus be roughly 1:320. However, this too would be misleading. Canterbury being the county town, its practitioners included men of high reputation who catered for an area much wider than six miles from the city (*see* chapter 4). Thus it can be seen that simple ratios of urban practitioners to urban populations are an imperfect way of estimating medical availability in any given place. It might be a valid exercise for a whole region – and a more accurate estimate of the ratio for the diocese will be attempted in chapter 3 – but not for a town or city in isolation.

To summarise, the relationship between medical consumption and urban settlements in East Kent is a complicated one on account of the great differences which existed in the nature and purposes of the various towns. To live within or very close to Canterbury or one of the handful of towns which had a large number of medical practitioners significantly increased the chances that, near death, medical help would be obtained, especially before the Interregnum. However, for those places at a distance from these six towns, several other smaller towns acted as channels through which medical services might be obtained, either by travel to the town or by requesting the attendance of a local practitioner. After the Interregnum practitioners settling in the smaller towns and rural parishes greatly increased the medical coverage of the diocese, so that probably no parish can be described as medically remote in 1690, however rural its outlook, and even the poorer sections of the community represented in these accounts – i.e. the non-destitute poor – were able to obtain medical relief in the furthest-flung places. Indeed, it would appear that the disparity of medical help in emergencies between medical towns and rural areas had by this time largely broken down, so that some rural areas were as well-served as the more established urban centres. This contrasts greatly with the very low levels of medical care afforded the dying in certain rural areas in Elizabethan times. Whether the initial low levels were primarily due to attitudes to medical intervention in providential matters, or the availability of expertise, or both, it is fair to say that the extraordinary growth in medical assistance to the dying in East Kent over the course of the seventeenth century is most noticeable in rural parishes. By 1690 medical practitioners were often resident in those remote areas where they had rarely even been employed a hundred years earlier.

Geography: nursing services

Unlike medical services to the dying, nursing services show very little variation across region or distance from towns. For Status A and B, the proportion

to reflect the likely comparative populousness of villages in the hinterland of the county town: C. W. Chalklin, *Seventeenth century Kent: a social and economic history*, London 1965, 27.

of all accounts with nursing entries between 1570 and 1690 remained at 15–17 per cent for those within towns and at 12–17 per cent for those more than three miles away. For the lower status groups the proportion employing nurses was similarly 14–17 per cent for urban dwellers and a consistent 13–14 per cent for those more than three miles from town. The only surprising point about these figures is that the level of nursing care in the rural areas – where there was a 'medical disadvantage' – was not greater than in towns. The explanation is probably to be found in the aspect of charging for nursing care; it could be that nursing services had to be paid for more regularly in towns than in rural areas.

The one area where there was an area of change was in the exclusive use of nursing help, without medicine (*see* tables 2–5). This was not a choice or development which bore any relation to urban or rural location. Although in all areas widows and spinsters more frequently employed a nursing-only strategy in their last sickness, there was no geographical disparity between the urban and the rural use of paid nurses exclusive of medical help. The vast majority of helpers, keepers, nurses, watchers, tenders and attendants were local women experienced in tending the sick and dying, whether urban or rural.

Table 15
Nursing care without medical help in relation to medical towns

Distance	A, B males		C, D males		All females	
	<1 mile %	>3 miles %	<1 mile %	>3 miles %	<1 mile %	>3 miles %
1570–99	11	14	11	12	23	12
1600–29	6	8	9	11	20	21
1630–49	3	7	9	10	15	15
1660–89	6	3	7	6	9	8
1690–1719	1	4	5	3	12	11

Note: All figures are percentages of all accounts for that status group in that proximity, not just those with medical and nursing entries.

The model of medical services in East Kent is a complex but coherent one. Even as early as 1570 there was a trickle of medical assistance available to all seriously ill and dying people, including the poor, and in all areas of the county, not just the towns. However, the proportion of those who took up a medical strategy to cope with their life-threatening condition was very small. Prior to 1600, the vast majority of people of all classes opted for nursing care to alleviate their suffering more often than medical practitioners. Higher status patients more frequently purchased medicine than their less well-off contemporaries, but only slightly more. Similarly, urban dwellers more often opted for medical strategies than their rural counterparts, but not to a very great extent. But all these groups took part in a huge social shift towards medical solutions to life-threatening problems between 1610 and 1670. Increasingly all the inhabitants of the region – whether they were urban, rural, rich or not-so-rich – sought out and employed practitioners in and from the key medical towns. The highest status group increased its propensity to pay for medicine by 400 per cent between the late sixteenth century and the start of the eighteenth. Status B increased the regularity of their medical consumption by 550 per cent, Status C by about 1,400 per cent and Status D by over 1,000 per cent. Nor was this just an urban phenomenon; rural low-status patients saw a 1,130 per cent growth in their adoption of medical strategies over the period. Even if the data after 1690 is considered too partial to be wholly reliable, it is clear that rural lower status patients experienced an increase in medicine of about 520 per cent in the period from about 1585 to 1675 (see appendix). These huge increases cannot be described as anything but a profound shift in attitude towards medicine on the part of the seriously ill and dying. By the end of the period under investigation more dying people of all status groups were obtaining medical help in the last days and weeks of life than were not. Nursing remained a relatively constant form of employment for urban and rural women, but the proportion of people paying for nursing care only, and not bothering with medicine, had dwindled by 1700 to a negligible level.

How does this correlate with what was previously known of medical strategies in the face of severe illness? The idea that most of England was medically remote in the seventeenth century cannot now be regarded as correct; only at the start of the seventeenth century were the remotest areas of East Kent beyond the regular reach of medical practitioners. The turn-around from a nursing strategy to a medical one has, moreover, been heralded in other areas of writing. Those who have worked extensively on the role of spiritual physic have emphasised its importance at the start, but not at the end, of the seventeenth century.[38] Around 1600 the widespread use of exclusively nursing strategies is consistent with a population which largely turned to God or 'Christ the Physician' when facing severe illness. The analysis of the probate accounts supports the decline of this belief. Thus, although the applications for diocesan medical licences in the 1660s very often stress the practitioner's religious credentials, and the purity of his life, such references soon disappear from these documents so that, by the end of the seventeenth century, the practitioner's medical education is more important than his morality. By the late seventeenth century widely differing views of the importance of religion

---

[38] For spiritual physic see D. Harley, 'Spiritual physic, providence and English medicine', in O. P. Grell and A. Cunningham (eds), Medicine and the Reformation, London 1993, 101–17; A. Wear, 'Puritan perceptions of illness in seventeenth century England', in R. Porter (ed.), Patients and practitioners: lay perceptions of medicine in pre-industrial society, Cambridge 1985, 55–100; and A. Wear, 'Religious beliefs and medicine in early modern England', in H. Marland and M. Pelling (eds), The task of healing, Rotterdam 1996, 146–69.

to healing were being espoused. Roy Porter has provided evidence for this, contrasting Ralph Josselin's view that his family's illnesses were a providential matter with Pepys, who understood his illnesses in purely secular and medical terms.[39] Similarly contrasting views can be found in the diaries of Bulstrode Whitelocke and Ralph Josselin. Providence still had a part to play in attitudes to early eighteenth-century bouts of illness (as may be seen in the diary of Richard Kay for example) but it was not nearly so widely seen as the best course of action.[40] Clearly the view that God would aid the sufferer – and that no other help was needed – was breaking down over the course of the seventeenth century, and an increased tendency among patients to take matters into their own hands was a part of this breakdown. In this sense the probate account statistics for East Kent confirm and provide a measurement of what many social historians have long suspected.

[39] D. Porter and R. Porter, *Patients' progress: doctors and doctoring in eighteenth-century England*, Oxford 1989, 5.
[40] R. Houlbrooke, *Death, religion and the family in England, 1480–1750*, Oxford 1998, 184–5.

2

The Medicalisation of Central
Southern England

How relevant is the East Kent model to the rest of provincial southern England? This is a difficult question to answer. In theory it should be easy – a direct comparison between dioceses using the same methods – but in practice this is not possible. No other county has a collection of accounts which compares in size with that of Kent, and thus no other county can be examined in the same detail per decade as East Kent. Nor is any other collection of accounts as detailed in its medical references. Even a cursory glance at the index for other regions shows that the entries denoting medical assistance and sickness are not nearly as common for other counties as they are for East Kent.

The records of diocesan licensing also suggest that we should not expect medical services to be directly comparable across regions. In the period 1570–1649 no fewer than 31 per cent of the East Kent practitioners named in the Canterbury probate accounts were diocesan licentiates. This is a surprisingly high figure, as current thinking is that relatively few medical practitioners had a degree or a licence.[1] For accounts dating to the period 1660–1719 the proportion was even higher, at 39 per cent. Such figures naturally lead to suspicions that the clerks writing the accounts tended only to name ecclesiastically licensed practitioners. It is more likely, however, that current thinking needs to be revised, with regard to East Kent at least, for not only were licentiates more frequently named in the probate accounts, they were also more common on the ground in Kent than is normally stated. In the diocese of Canterbury there were four to six times as many practitioners with diocesan licences per head of the population as there were in the dioceses of Exeter, Salisbury, Lincoln and Chichester.

This immediately demonstrates why any generalisation about medical assistance to the dying in southern England based solely on Kent records is open to question. Most counties seem to have had a diocesan medical licentiate-to-population ratio of about 1:4,000. Even if the highest multipliers suggested for population figures derived from the Compton Census are employed, the population of the diocese of Canterbury was hardly any

1   Pelling and Webster, 'Medical practitioners', 193.

Table 16
Diocesan-licensed practitioner: population ratios for East Kent, Devon and Cornwall, and Wiltshire*

| | East Kent (c. 76,000) | | Devon and Cornwall (c. 330,000) | | Wiltshire (c. 120,000) | |
	Dioc. lic.	Ratio	Dioc. lic.	Ratio	Dioc. lic.	Ratio
1610–49	91	1:830	86	1:3840	n/k	n/k
1660–89	126	1:600	83	1:3980	19	1:6320
1690–1719	65	1:1160	78	1:4230	28	1:4290

Note: Figures in brackets are population estimates for the period 1660–76

* Ratios given to the nearest 10. The population of East Kent is derived from P. Brandon and B. Short, *The south east from AD 1000*, London 1990, 190–6; that of Devon and Cornwall is from J. Barry, 'Population distribution and growth in the early modern period', in R. Kain and W. Ravenhill (eds), *Historical atlas of south-west England*, Exeter 1999, 116–17, and 'South-west' in P. Clark (ed.), *The Cambridge urban history of Britain*, II: *1540–1840*, Cambridge 2000, 67–92 at p. 68, where that of Wiltshire also appears. A rough check on Wiltshire can be run by multiplying the 1801 census figure (185,107, according to E. A. Wrigley and R. Schofield, *The population history of England, 1841–1871*, London 1981, 622) by the differential between the national back-projection figures for 1660 and 1801 (5.13 million / 8.66 million, according to Wrigley and Schofield, ibid. 532–4); rounding to the nearest 5,000 gives 110,000. Numbers of licentiates have been taken from the Wellcome Trust Library, London, MS 5343. Chalklin suggests that the population of Kent as a whole was fairly static over the seventeenth century, perhaps rising from 130,000 to 150,000 between 1600 and 1676: *Seventeenth century Kent*, 27.

more than 100,000, which would give ratios of 1:790 to 1:1,540.[2] The presence of four times as many diocesan licentiates per head of the population in Kent, coupled with plentiful evidence of their activity, has two particular implications. Medical assistance in East Kent was very probably organised much more strictly according to licensing legislation than in other counties, perhaps through a greater level of rigour with regard to visitations. And it is possible – although in no way certain – that Kent benefited from a greater number of practitioners serving the dying, not just a greater number of licentiates.

[2] T. Arkell, 'A method for estimating population totals from the Compton Census returns', in K. Schurer and T. Arkell (eds), *Surveying the people: the interpretation and use of document sources for the study of population in the later seventeenth century*, Oxford 1992, 97–116. The multiplying range suggested is from 1.4 to 1.7: the Compton Census total for East Kent is 59,654. Working on the basis that the total population was approximately four times the number of houses specified in the 1690 Hearth Books (which tallies with these estimates for Berkshire, Sussex and Wiltshire), then the population of both East and West Kent was in the region of 190,000, East Kent being about half of this.

Table 17
Diocesan-licensed practitioner: population ratios for Sussex, Berkshire and the diocese of Lincoln*

	Diocese of Lincoln (c. 260,000)		Sussex (c. 90,000)		Berkshire (c. 65,000)	
	Dioc. lic.	Ratio	Dioc. lic.	Ratio	Dioc. lic.	Ratio
1610–49	n/k	–	n/k	–	n/k	–
1660–89	51	1:5100	24?	1:3750	n/k	–
1690–1719	46	1:5650	n/k	–	17?	1:3820

Note: Figures in brackets are population estimates for the period 1660–76

* Ratios given to the nearest 10. The 1660–89 figure for the diocese of Lincoln is based on there being thirty-three recorded entries in the subscription book (which begins in 1670) for the period 1670–89. The population figures have been obtained as follows: For Sussex and Berkshire the figures have been derived in the same way as for Wiltshire, by multiplying the 1801 census figure by the differential between the national back-projection figures for 1660 and 1801, and rounding to the nearest 5,000. This gives 95,000 for Sussex and 65,000 for Berkshire. Since Barry's estimates for Devon and Cornwall and Wiltshire are roughly 1.5 times the Compton Census figures (adults) given in *Compton Census*, pp. cx-cxi, and so are Chalklin's figures for Kent, a second rough check is possible by multiplying the county figures given in Whiteman by 1.5. This gives 90,000 for Sussex (East and West) and 65,000 for Berkshire. The two methods do not tally however, when trying to estimate figures for the diocese of Lincolnshire. Back-projection on each county suggests c.225,000 and calculations based on a multiple of 1.5 of Whiteman's figures suggest 300,000. A rough average of 260,000 has been used, in view of the absence of any more accurate figures. Numbers of licentiates have been taken from Wellcome Trust Library, London, MSS 5343–7 (A. W. G. Haggis, typescript list of medical licentiates).

With these *caveats* in mind the probate records of the counties of central southern England, namely Berkshire, Wiltshire and West Sussex may be analysed. Immediately there is a methodological problem; these collections were not indexed by the same person as the East Kent collections. There are many fewer index entries relating to medical assistance and illnesses. Close examination of a sample of the documents shows that, although the index does not ignore all nursing entries in Sussex or Berkshire (as many of these appear in the same documents as medical entries), it does so with such regularity that it cannot be used to quantify nursing in these counties.[3] So the only way to check the relevance of the East Kent model of medicalisation for these counties is with respect to medical assistance.

The figures in table 18 might be taken as an indication that East Kent enjoyed significantly more medical assistance than the other counties in the later seventeenth century. However, a number of factors must be considered before leaping to such a conclusion. First, there should be a strong suspi-

[3] Mortimer, 'Medical assistance', i. 132–3.

Table 18
Accounts with medical-related entries in relation to total extant accounts

Date	East Kent %	Berkshire %	West Sussex %	Wiltshire %
1570–99	5	10	3	–
1600–29	8	6	8	3
1630–49	15	6	5	3
1660–89	27	12	20	11

Note: This does not include references to nursing

cion that the diocese of Canterbury, which took the creation of probate accounts so seriously that it made many more accounts *per capita* than any other region, also took the inclusion of detail with as great a seriousness. East Kent accounts are much fuller than those for the diocese of Salisbury. That the most thorough application of the ecclesiastical medical licensing system took place within the same jurisdiction as arguably the most thorough application of the probate law is probably not a coincidence, and the same institutional conscience may have guided the Canterbury clerks to enquire more fully into medical practitioners' involvement than elsewhere.[4]

A second reason not to presume that medicine was more commonly obtained in East Kent may be discerned by closely examining the different characteristics of the accounts from different courts. This is clearest in two dozen Wiltshire accounts for which drafts are extant: medical references have been edited by the clerk, who wrapped payments for watching, tending and physic up in the same entry as 'funeral charges'. For example, the draft account of John Hayes (d. 1684) has three medical and nursing entries: 'to Hester Harding who attended him in his sicknesse for her attendance 14s; for the physicion in his sicknesse 15s; To the Apothecary & messengers 1s 4d'. In the final version this appears as: 'Inprimis this Accomptant craveth Allowance of £3 4s 7d being necessarily expended in the sicknesse of the deceased & in his funeralls & all other necessaryes thereto belonging'.[5] Nor is this a one-off case: Wiltshire accounts are frequently vague, referring to 'expenses in his sickness'. This prevents a researcher from indexing the account in relation to medical practice or sickness. Although such condensing of medical details happened less frequently in Sussex, where payments for medical help were often recorded in a different 'petitions' section rather than under 'funeral expenses', it was noticed in the course of systematically examining a series of Chichester documents that some proper names were

4 Idem, 'Why were probate accounts made?', 2–17.
5 WRO, P3/H/625

frequently repeated. 'Paid to Mr Peachey' is a good example; it was only later – after laying aside many such apparently non-medical accounts – that a fuller description was found: 'paid to Mr Peachey the Chirurgion'.

As a result the process of assimilating data about medical assistance to the dying must be considered as a multi-layered filtration process in each diocese or archdeaconry. At the first level of filtration there was the drawing up of the draft account. This was done in a number of ways: in some cases accountants, interested only in the disbursement of assets, did not bother to record all payments. Minor payments to practitioners or nurses may have been neglected by those who regarded them as trifling sums and who were more interested in large amounts of money owed on bond or desperate debts. The second level of filtration was the court's assimilation of payments from the draft and the accountant and presenting them in its 'house style'. In some courts this meant condensing information into totals and cutting out as much detail as possible; in Sussex it meant that medical payments might be left as debts or 'petitions' of an unspecified nature. Berkshire documents tend to be the briefest of all, and might incorporate both the above features. Many Sussex accounts, in concentrating only on the distribution of the estates of solvent intestates, omitted all expenses except those of the court. In Kent, by contrast, the specific details of expenditure were normally included in full. At the third level of filtration there is the physical disruption to the document over the centuries. Many Sussex documents have lost headers and footers: this tends to eradicate information about sickness at certain periods when it appeared in the 'petitions' section, frequently at the top of the second side of the folio. The fourth and final level of filtration is the inconsistent interpretation of the subject-indexing procedure, especially with regard to nursing.

The end result of these filtration processes is an index composed of three or four datasets which cannot be used to compare actual levels of involvement – whether nursing or medical – across separate ecclesiastical jurisdictions. But although direct comparison of levels of medical involvement is impossible, in those regions where the processes described above acted as a filter rather than an inhibitor on the recording of medicine and sickness, it is possible to compare rates of change. Hence the changes within each county may be examined to see whether the significant increase in the use of medical services in East Kent was unique at this period or was experienced elsewhere.

To assess the comparative rates of change, the proportions of dying men and women of middling wealth (£40–£200) receiving medical assistance have been compared across the four counties. Insufficient documents survive from the sixteenth and eighteenth centuries, so the date ranges compared are only for the seventeenth. Nevertheless, the figures (see table 19) reveal a significant increase in the use of medicine in all the counties.

The samples in these respective counties may be assumed to have as many people of higher status falling into the middling wealth band as each other,

Table 19
Increments in the proportion of males and females with estates
of value £40–£200 receiving medical assistance

Date range	East Kent	Berkshire	West Sussex	Wiltshire
A: 1600–29	9%	6%	7%	3%
B: 1630–49	16%	8%	6%	3%
C: 1660–89	27%	12%	18%	9%
Increments				
B/A	1.70	1.28	0.89	0.89
C/A	2.85	1.93	2.56	2.79

Note: The increments have been worked out on the actual figures, not the rounded percentages

and therefore are directly comparable (with the exception of damage to some of the West Sussex documents). The substantial increases noted in East Kent are almost matched in Wiltshire and West Sussex. Berkshire, with a rise of just 93 per cent in the reported use of medicine, was the least medically changed region. While the increments over the first half of the period suggest little or no change in Wiltshire and Sussex, perhaps even a slight fall, it appears that the extraordinary increases in the use of medicine found in all East Kent status groups in the mid-seventeenth century are symptomatic not merely of a local change but of one which had embraced much if not all of provincial southern England by 1690, and probably other regions too. This is possibly the reason for similar rises in the probate account collections of other dioceses at this time.[6] On the basis of verified data, it may be said, with some conviction, that between the reigns of James I and James II the tendency for people of middling wealth to obtain medical assistance doubled, and in some places tripled, in central southern England as well as in East Kent.

Wealth and status

This argument demonstrates a widespread increase in the number of medical assistance payments on behalf of those of middling wealth. Was this the case for all status groups? The next question demanding attention is whether the status-related variations in Kent were similar to those in other counties, or whether greater or smaller variations in the propensity to pay for medical assistance may be noted.

---

6   Mortimer, 'Medical assistance', ii. 37–8.

Table 20
Increments in the proportion of higher status groups receiving medical assistance

Date	East Kent	Berkshire	West Sussex	Wiltshire
A: 1600–29	13%	6%	12%	5%
B: 1630–49	20%	7%	9%	5%
C: 1660–89	31%	14%	21%	16%
Increments				
B/A	1.52	1.05	0.74	1.06
C/A	2.39	2.15	1.83	3.45

Note: Status groups A, B and R as defined in chapter 1 (males and females). Increments have been worked out on the actual figures, not the rounded percentages.

Table 21
Increments in the proportion of lower status groups receiving medical assistance

Date	East Kent	Berkshire	West Sussex	Wiltshire
A: 1600–29	7%	6%	6%	2.5%
B: 1630–49	13%	5%	3%	3%
C: 1660–89	23%	10%	18%	7%
Increments				
B/A	1.96	0.91	0.52	1.12
C/A	3.52	1.76	2.88	2.83

Note: Status groups C, D and S as defined in chapter 1 (males and females). Increments have been worked out on the actual figures, not the rounded percentages.

This question raises a fundamental methodological problem. For Wiltshire there is only one Status A account for the period 1570–99; for Berkshire there are only twenty; for Sussex there are only nine. Statements of worth cannot be made on the strength of so few documents. One option is to examine the central southern area as a whole, but this does not remedy the lack of documents for the early period and, moreover, it ignores the significant problem of comparing information which has been through separate filtration processes. An alternative option is to extend the periods under examination, for example to examine trends in Status A patients from 1570 to 1649 compared to 1660 to 1719; this however prevents any real sense of temporal definition. It also ignores the fact that lower status accounts are common prior to the Civil Wars and comparatively scarce after the Restoration, while higher status accounts are comparatively scarce in the earlier period and common in the later one. Nor can customised date periods for each county be drawn up and the comparability of the data be preserved. The best solution is to select two groups for further comparative analysis in each county between 1600 and 1690: Status A and B men together with Status R women; and Status C and D men together with Status S women.

While we might labour to explain the apparent declines and discrepancies through changing practices in each diocesan and archdeaconry court, such efforts would miss the main point. The C/A (c. 1675/c. 1615) ratio in all the counties indicates a substantial shift towards medical strategies throughout central southern England. When it is recalled that the increments noted for East Kent are representative of changes in excess of 1,000 per cent for the lower status groups over the whole period (from 1570), and 400–500 per cent for the higher ones, the comparability is striking. The statistics leave no room to doubt that central southern England experienced changes similar to those described for East Kent.

With regard to extent of the process of medicalisation, the Wiltshire higher status groups seem to have increased their take-up of medical assistance to an even greater level than their contemporaries in East Kent. Their lower status neighbours, like those in West Sussex, saw increases almost as substantial as East Kent. Where these three counties all differ from East Kent is in the matter of when these changes took place. Although the shift was well under way in East Kent by 1649, no significant increases in medical assistance are to be noted in the other three counties at that time. In fact, central southern England seems to have been about twenty to thirty years behind East Kent in adopting medical strategies on behalf of the dying, and Wiltshire seems to have been slowest of all. It was not until after the Interregnum that the process of medicalisation in central southern England noticeably occurred.

Gender

Due to the small number of accounts made for women outside Kent, and the necessity of dividing this number in order to concentrate upon women of comparable status in the various counties, it is not possible to have much confidence in a test on the higher status individuals except in East Kent. However, rather than simply ignore the question of whether there was a close correlation between the propensity of females and males outside East Kent to receive medical help, a test has been run in which lower status – Status S – females across all three sample counties have been compared with Status C and D males in each county (see table 22). From this it appears that the close comparison observed in East Kent was even closer in other counties. When the need struck, women were just as prepared as men to receive medical help from male practitioners.

Table 22
Proportions of lower status males and females obtaining medical help

Date	East Kent		Wiltshire, Berkshire, West Sussex	
Status	S	C, D	S	C, D
	%	%	%	%
1600–29	9	6	5	5
1630–49	13	13	5	4
1660–89	24	23	9	11

Geography: medical services

As with gender-related distinctions, the relatively small numbers of accounts for the central southern counties mean that the same searching methods as for East Kent cannot be applied. In addition, whereas it was possible to build up a detailed listing of the medical practitioners in East Kent from a large number of sources, not the least of which are the licensing records, it is not possible to do the same for the other counties. Berkshire, West Sussex and Wiltshire licensing records are relatively few and incomplete. Similarly their accounts only rarely include the names and towns of medical practitioners. As a result, it is not possible to identify medical towns in the same way as was done for East Kent, nor is it possible to check the 'loyalty' of residents in the hinterland of any given town when requiring medical assistance. Having said this, there are ways to test the East Kent model, although different techniques need to be used to decide what constituted a medical town, and a lower threshold of accounts must be used to investigate changes over time.

Berkshire

Using the same authorities used for determining Kent towns – John Norden's *An intended guyde for English travaillers* (1625) and (Anon) *A book of the names of all parishes, market towns, villages, hamlets* (1662) – a list of 'towns' for Berkshire can be drawn up. The lists agree with one another: Abingdon, Faringdon, Hungerford, East Ilsley, Lambourn, Maidenhead, Newbury, Reading, Wallingford, Wantage, Windsor and Wokingham. If they are compared with Everitt's list of markets probably active about 1600, the lists correlate. Although it is not possible to establish which of these might have been considered a medical town under the same criteria as for East Kent, most Kentish medical towns appeared on these lists for 1625 and 1662. If Oxford is added as the obvious other medical town, as it is on the northern tip of Berkshire, then a list of thirteen might be considered satisfactory. Joan Dils, however, in her chapter on 'Berkshire towns, 1500–1700', excludes

Table 23
Urban bias of Berkshire medical accounts: all status groups

Date	<1 mile %	1–3 miles %	>3 miles %
1600–49	16	5	5
1660–89	11	12	12

Lambourn and East Ilsley.[7] Lambourn was not a very populous place, and is itself somewhat remote, but its neighbouring parishes are all at least partly within six miles of another town on the lists. Thus, following Dils, this location has been ignored as probably of no more than minor importance in economic terms, and even less as a medical centre. East Ilsley on the other hand, although its importance might have been just as slight, has not been completely ignored, as several parishes within its six-mile hinterland are not within such a distance of another town. It has thus been regarded in the same way as Lenham in East Kent: as a potential medical focus for those parishes which are more than six miles from other towns. The result is a series of twelve 'towns', including Oxford, which between them leave only one parish in the north of the county more than six miles from a town (Longworth) and a narrow band of parishes between east and west Berkshire. These – Basildon, Beenham, Bradfield, Padworth, Pangbourne, Shaw cum Donnington, Sulhampstead Abbots, Upton Nervet and Woolhampton – all lie entirely outside a six-mile radius of the nearest town.

Table 23 suggests that in Berkshire, as in East Kent, geographical relationship to a town was a factor in determining use of medical services in the period prior to the Interregnum. After 1660 the disparity between rural and urban medical assistance disappeared. This is interesting because, of all the sample counties, the discrepancy between higher and lower status use of medicine was at its slightest in Berkshire, and was closely comparable with Kent after the Restoration.[8] Thus any status bias inadvertently introduced into the table through rural/urban polarisation should be minimal. It follows that what is being seen here is the closest that can be achieved to a pure geographical test of the East Kent model; and like Kent it seems that any medical disadvantage to rural living, although distinct in the sixteenth century, had disappeared by 1690.

This is not to imply that there were no medically remote areas in Berkshire. To test this medical payments in Reading may be compared with the nine parishes which fall between east and west Berkshire towns, more than six miles on either side, a process which suggests that the medical disad-

[7] J. Dils, 'Berkshire towns, 1500–1700', in J. Dils (ed.), *An historical map of Berkshire* (Berkshire Record Society, 1998), 50–1.
[8] Mortimer, 'Medical assistance', i. 139.

Table 24
Medical assistance in remote parishes compared with major towns

Date	<2 miles from Reading %	<2 miles from A., N., or W. %	Remote %
1600–49	23	8	6
1660–89	15	15	12

Note: A = Abingdon; N. = Newbury; W = Wallingford. Remote refers to parishes more than six miles from a medical town. Data includes both sexes, all status groups.

vantage of living in these remote parishes was most marked prior to the Interregnum. Having said this, the figures for Abingdon, Newbury and Wallingford suggest that this was not so much because of the remoteness of these nine parishes as Reading's pre-eminence as a medical town at that time. Afterwards, as in East Kent, the rural disadvantage was minimal.

West Sussex

West Sussex also has an easily definable set of towns. Norden's *Intended guyde* (1625) and the anonymous *Names of all parishes* (1662) both suggest Arundel, Chichester, Horsham, Midhurst, Petworth, Shoreham, Steyning and (West) Tarring. While the last of these is a doubtful medical town, being described as 'decayed', there is no doubting the importance of the others as local or regional centres. Everitt notes all of them, including West Tarring, as market towns in about 1600, plus Storrington which was 6.5 miles from Arundel.[9] Five of these eight towns actually appear as 'hometowns' of practitioners noted in the twenty-one accounts which give such details. Almost the whole of West Sussex (the archdeaconry of Chichester) falls within six miles of the five – Arundel, Chichester, Horsham, Midhurst and Petworth – or Steyning. The parishes of Compton, Stoughton and Up Marden in the far west are all partly beyond the six miles from Chichester but come within six miles of Petersfield in Hampshire. The only other parishes in the whole archdeaconry which predominantly lie more than six miles beyond one of these six towns are Selsey, West Chiltington and Goring, the latter two each being about seven miles from several towns. Parishes on the fringes of the county such as Linchmere are near towns in Surrey and Hampshire (Haslemere in the case of Linchmere). Thus there is every reason to regard Sussex as more evenly spread with towns than the other counties being studied.

Table 25 reveals a distinct difference between urban and rural tendencies to obtain medical help after the Restoration, in contrast to the findings for

[9]   A. Everitt, 'Market towns, c. 1500–1640', in J. Thirsk (ed.), *The agrarian history of England and Wales*, iv, Cambridge 1967, 466–589 at p. 475.

52

Table 25
Urban bias of West Sussex medical accounts: all status groups

Date	<1 mile %	1–3 miles %	>3 miles %
1600–49	12	4	11
1660–89	34	18	17

Berkshire and East Kent. The medical advantage of urban living in both East Kent and Berkshire was minimal after the Restoration but in West Sussex it persisted after 1660, despite almost all the archdeaconry being within easy reach of a town. Although the sample sizes are not as large as might be hoped (the smallest, yielding the 34 per cent figure, is sixty-one documents), it would appear that medical assistance remained more focused within towns in West Sussex than in Berkshire and Kent after 1660.

Wiltshire

Wiltshire is a far more complicated case. The very question of what constitutes a medical town is impossible to establish with any great confidence. Norden in his 1625 list included several seats, coaching towns and other places which cannot be considered towns without diluting the sample of 'towns' beyond meaning. The 1662 list gives seventeen towns, but again some of these are doubtful.[10] Albourne and Wootton Bassett, for example, cannot be connected with any degree of medical assistance in the eighteenth century, let alone in the seventeenth. The 1686 list of places for accommodation (drawn up with the billeting of troops in mind) does not tally very well with the 1662 list: only eleven places appear on both.[11] Everitt's list of markets active about 1600 gives no fewer than twenty-three places which, if all were indeed active, include some very minor market towns. A generation earlier, the 1576 subsidy for Wiltshire describes only eight places as 'borough' and three as 'town'. While a list of towns could be taken from another source, this would not constitute a likely list of medical towns (as opposed to wool, coaching or market towns). Unfortunately the medical licensing records for the diocese are poor and of limited use in furnishing a list of medical centres. The probate accounts are similarly limited in describing practitioners' places of residence.

---

10 These are: Albourne, Amesbury, Bradford, Calne, Castle Combe, Chippenham, Cricklade, Devizes, Highworth, Lavington, Malmesbury, Marlborough, Salisbury, Trowbridge, Westbury, Wilton and Wootton Bassett.
11 N. J. Williams, *Tradesmen in early Stuart Wiltshire*, Devizes 1960, p. xv: list of towns with stabling and beds (quoting WO 30/48).

The best that can be done is to use those places described as certainly towns and compare those within the near and far hinterlands, adding the major medical towns just beyond the border: Hungerford (Berks), Bath (Somerset) and Shaftesbury (Dorset), and their hinterlands. This gives the following towns in addition to those outside Wiltshire: Amesbury, Bradford, Calne, Chippenham, Cricklade, Devizes, Malmesbury, Marlborough, Salisbury, Trowbridge and Wilton. To maximise the number of accounts which fall within these areas, the 1–3 miles and 3+ miles hinterlands have been pooled. This reveals that, in the fifty years 1600–49, the level of medical help purchased was roughly comparable in town and six-mile hinterland: about 3 per cent. After 1660 the level of medical help purchased on behalf of the dying by town-dwellers in Wiltshire increased dramatically, to 17 per cent, and in the rural hinterland more than doubled, to over 8 per cent. It is interesting that the removal of all Status A men from this latter calculation shows that there was virtually no increase in the hinterland regions: the medicalisation of rural Wiltshire was led by the rich.

This test ignores swathes of rural Wiltshire, including probably the most remote parts of the county, and this remains a weakness of the findings. Nevertheless the results are significant, for focusing on just these towns and their hinterlands reveals the possibility of very substantial growth – of the order of 400 per cent in the towns compared to an almost stagnant medical situation among the less well-off only a mile or two away. Wiltshire seems to have experienced growth in the use of medicine much later than Berkshire, West Sussex and East Kent, and only in urban settlements. Amongst the less well-off perhaps five times as many townsmen as countrymen obtained medicine. The evidence suggests that in Wiltshire alone of the four counties geography was a critical factor in obtaining medical help in the post-Restoration period. Once the growth in medical assistance developed it seems to have remained an urban phenomenon until at least 1680–90, whereas in East Kent and Berkshire it spread out to the hinterlands well before the penultimate decade of the century.

There is no doubt that central southern England increasingly adopted medical strategies in the same way as in East Kent. Although it is not possible directly to compare the levels of medical care taken from different processes of creating evidence, the comparable levels of change show that every county saw huge increases over the third quarter of the seventeenth century, continuing a trend which was noticeable in East Kent from twenty or thirty years earlier. The delay is perhaps surprising. So too is the discovery that there were so many more licensed practitioners in East Kent. Indeed, comparing East Kent and rural Wiltshire presents the most startling contrasts: Kent was experiencing rapid medicalisation in all status groups and all areas by 1650, with nowhere being left medically remote, whereas Wiltshire was comparatively backward, and the medicalisation process underway was exclusively enjoyed by urban and high-status families.

Table 26
Increases in payments for medical care between 1600–49 and 1660–89 in relation to status and residence

	Urban high status %	Urban lower status %	1–6 miles high status %	1–6 miles lower status %
East Kent	60	120	110	220
West Sussex	[100]	[250]	110	250
Berkshire	[120]	–50	100	170
Wiltshire	[530]	400	100	0

Note: High status = status groups A, B and R; Lower status = status groups C, D and S. Figures in square brackets are based on samples of fewer than fifty accounts. See appendix for full details.

The one anomaly, observable in table 26 – an apparent decline in the use of medical strategies by the less well-off in Berkshire – might be due to changing court procedure: summarising documents rather than specifying all the expenses. As this particular percentage is based on just fifty-one documents, it is impossible to be certain, but it is possible that the urban lower status groups started from a higher level of medical involvement than the other counties and thus lost out as urban practitioners increasingly served the rural hinterlands. What is not in doubt is that the rural well-off in every county were at least twice as likely to follow a medical strategy in the period 1660–89 as they were in the first half of the seventeenth century. Their less well-off contemporaries were even more likely to do so, usually starting from a lower level of medicalisation. Only Wiltshire stands outside this pattern, the rural poor experiencing no noticeable change with regard to medical services before 1690.

How can these differences be explained? There were probably cultural reasons for the medical advancement of East Kent. Of the four counties under investigation Kent as a whole was the most heavily settled, with forty-seven houses per thousand acres in 1690 (compared to thirty-six in Berkshire, thirty-one in Wiltshire and twenty-five in Sussex).[12] The customary division of land in East Kent – gavelkind – meant that the Kentish yeoman was a more prosperous, independent figure than the tenant farmers of central southern England. East Kent also stood astride the lines of communication between London, Canterbury, Dover and the continent: hence the number of resident Dutch, French and Jewish medical practitioners. But the most important reason is probably connected with practitioner availability and proximity to patients (see chapter 3).

[12] These figures have been derived from the 1690 Hearth Tax returns: *Seventeenth century economic documents*, ed. J. Thirsk and J. P. Cooper, Oxford 1972, 803.

On the basis of the figures presented in this chapter, it would appear that the East Kent model is indicative, rather than representative, of the growth in the use of medicine by the dying in the seventeenth century. The general trend was universal but it was followed in the other counties at slower rates, with people of different classes taking up the medical option at different times. Perhaps unsurprisingly, the most rural, the poorest and the least densely-populated areas were the slowest to do so. Although in all counties medical expertise was located in, or disseminated by way of, the larger urban settlements, and spread out from towns to the country, the rate of diffusion varied from place to place, in accordance with the geography and cultural links of the region. In East Kent the medical disadvantage of living in a rural area had all but disappeared by 1690; that is not something that can be said for the most rural areas of central southern England, in West Sussex and Wiltshire.

3

The Availability and Nature of Medical Assistance

If society was becoming medicalised, it follows that a group within it was acting – either consciously or unconsciously – as an agent for social change. It is reasonable to speculate that increases of several hundred per cent in medical services between the first and the third quarters of the seventeenth century led to a greater call on the time of practitioners, and so for a greater need for them. Was the ambition to be a medical practitioner partly behind the change? The supply-side factor is best measured by discovering whether there were more physicians, surgeons and apothecaries in 1690 than there had been at the start of the century. If there were, then this would be evidence of an increase in the use of medicine being common to all the sick, not just the seriously ill. It would also be evidence of the medicalisation of the county being driven by the medical practitioners themselves: their selling the idea of medical strategies to the population at large. Hence the first question to be answered in explaining how society became medicalised is whether it resulted in dramatic increases in the numbers of practitioners available.

Practitioner numbers

There are a number of ways in which to determine practitioner numbers. All the known names and dates of practitioners can be checked and thereby an absolute minimum established; but this method would permit very little scope systematically to assess how many practitioners are omitted from the records. A crude calculation based on the number of practitioners who were qualified, licensed, known to be active or had died in the space of one generation of about thirty years could be performed. For example, in East Kent in the period 1660–89 there were 263 practitioners known from some record or other, which, assuming a population of approximately 80,000 in 1676, suggests a ratio of 1:300 for the diocese. But this too is unsatisfactory, for by including all practitioners qualified and dying within the period, the number working or alive at any given time or in the space of a generation is not quantified, but rather anyone who began or ended his career, or died, in this period. The method used by Pelling and Webster to determine the numbers of London practitioners available in 1600, based on the total numbers of practitioners belonging to a Society or Company, is not possible in East Kent. There are no such companies covering rural areas or multiple towns.

The methodological approach which seems most satisfactory in the context of the data available is to estimate the numbers of practitioners by building a model of the career of each type of 'average practitioner' based on events in that career. Such events include the average period between licensing and death and between licensing and last activity as recorded in the probate accounts. In this way data may be rendered as practitioner-years, and these may in turn act as building blocks for an estimate of the number of practitioners in the diocese at a given date.

A good starting point is to consider the mean period between licensing and death (where approximate dates of death are known from grants of probate or compilation of probate inventories). Care must be taken to eliminate those whose dates of licensing were affected by the hiatus in diocesan licensing between 1643 and 1662 (a period which includes the glut after the dearth of licences granted). There are fifty practitioners for whom a date of death and a date of grant of licence are known. Excluding the fifteen who gained a licence immediately after the restoration of ecclesiastical authority (1661–2), their post-licensing lifespans range from one to fifty-three years.[1] From these it can be established that for this group the mean period of time between the granting of a medical licence and the practitioner's death was 21.8 years (median: 22 years). Of the fifteen practitioners who were licensed in the period 1661–2 (all diocesan) the post-licensing periods ranged from four to forty years, with a mean of 22.7 years (median: 26), which suggests that those who sought to obtain an ecclesiastical licence in 1661–2 were not necessarily men further advanced in their careers than if licensing had not been suspended. The mean is 22.3 years, or, including the one somewhat doubtful sixty-two-year post-licensing lifespan, 23.1 years. In the case of freemen of Canterbury there are only five definite accounts on which to work, but in these cases the length of time between receiving the freedom and death is not hugely different, at a mean of 26.4 years. These figures can be used partly to assess how many licensed and freemen practitioners were available at any given time. In a simple model, the number of licensed practitioners available in year 16XX would be roughly equivalent to all those to whom a licence was granted between [16XX – 22] and [16XX] inclusive (presuming a practitioner was able to practise in the year of his licensing, thus rounding the mean lifespan up to twenty-three years). To this figure may be added the freemen of Canterbury. If it is assumed that their post-freedom lifespan was in the region of twenty-six years, then likewise the number of freeman practitioners who might be expected to have been alive in year 16XX is measurable by establishing how many medically-related freedoms were awarded between [16XX – 25] and [16XX] inclusive.

---

[1] Mortimer, 'Medical assistance', ii. 44–5. A possible span of sixty-two years is that of Alexander Devison, but this might be two practitioners of the same name.

Table 27
Licentiate and freemen practitioners in East Kent

Date	Licensed practitioners	Canterbury freemen
1610	[n/a]	10 (+ 3 also licensed.)
1620	83	15 (+ 3 lic'd.)
1630	78	16 (+ 2 lic'd)
1640	82	19 (+ 5 lic'd)
1650	[n/a]	16 (+ 5 lic'd)
1660	[n/a]	11 (+4 lic'd)
1670	[95]	13 (+4 lic'd)
1680	[116]	21 (+3 lic'd)
1690	49	24 (0 lic'd)
1700	49	27 (0 lic'd)
1710	68	25 (+ 3 lic'd)
1720	57	21 (+5 lic'd)

Note: Licensed practitioners relates to those flourishing at any given time, based on a 23-year post-licensing lifespan; Canterbury freemen is based on a 26-year lifespan after becoming a freeman (excluding those who were also licentiates). Figures in square brackets are those affected by the hiatus in licensing. Unsuccessful applicants for licences have not been included.

This method is incomplete. As is well known, licentiates often practised for a period of time prior to licensing. Sometimes licence applications mention twenty or thirty years' experience, and while such long periods are not the norm, and have perhaps been exaggerated by the few writers who have commented upon applications for licences, this is not an insignificant matter.[2] However, it is very difficult to determine this period of time accurately. If all the pre-licensing appearances of the names of licentiates in the probate accounts were averaged out, this would create an artificially high figure, being based only on those cases in which pre-licensing was particularly marked. Similarly if a period of pre-licensing activity were averaged out across all the practitioners, this would result in an artificially low figure, for it would be based on the assumption that the pre-licensing cases identified in the accounts – very probably the minority – were the only cases of pre-licensing from the whole sample. It is possible to develop a more sophisticated methodology, extrapolating a period from the few known cases of pre-licensing medical payments.[3] However, the resultant minimum likely

[2]   Thus 'the most notable and common qualification is that [diocesan] applicants had "for many years practised the art"': Mortimer, 'Diocesan licensing', 61. See also John Guy, 'The episcopal licensing of physicians, surgeons and midwives', *Bulletin of the History of Medicine* lvi (1982), 528–42 at p. 534.
[3]   Mortimer, 'Medical assistance', ii. 51.

pre-licensing period of medical practice is wholly dependent on establishing a representative sample of the pre-licensing payments. This is not possible. Although some practitioners will have had twenty or so years experience prior to licensing, where such entries appear in the accounts there is rarely any justification for presuming that they are one and the same person. For example, Thomas Knowler, the physician active at Harbledown in 1681, may or may not have been the Thomas Knowler licensed to practise surgery at Canterbury in 1701. While it may well be that a more impressionistic figure would be more accurate, it is a contradiction in terms to give an impressionistic figure with accuracy: is three years or seven more accurate? It is just as difficult to determine how many years should be counted off the end of a career for an average period of retirement, or wind-down towards complete retirement (if practitioners ever did entirely give up physic). In view of these issues, a two-year period has been used, which is certainly an underestimate, but one which perhaps should not be extended in view of the possible number of retirements, or reduced working hours in old age.

Using this adjustment, the number of 'licensed practitioners' serving the dying (albeit some not yet licensed) at any given time may be quantified as those qualified between [16XX − 22] and [16XX + 2] inclusive. Only six Canterbury freemen are noted in the records as being paid for a medical service before they received their freedoms. These average 4.7 years earlier than freedom. It should be noted that a few practitioners (e.g. Robert Pemell) were granted their freedom as a reward for many years' service or fame, thereby increasing the probability that they would be described in the probate accounts prior to receiving their freedom. However, it would be wrong to base a judgement affecting all the freemen practitioners on the evidence of a few accounts, especially where those indicating pre-freedom experience are not the same as those indicating total post-freedom lifespan.

It is clear from the probate accounts that many practitioners were not licensed by the bishop or the archbishop, and nor were they freemen of Canterbury. They may have been degree-holders, even holders of medical degrees who did not have licences, failed applicants for licences, apprentices who did not serve out their whole term, freemen of a town other than Canterbury, licentiates of another body (e.g. the English universities or the College of Physicians) or practitioners unrecognised in any official capacity. These groups are much more difficult to quantify. However, it is possible to draw up a similar model of their lifespans comparable to the one constructed for licensing. Having done this, the proportions of licensed personnel appearing in the probate accounts can be calculated, and this proportion can be used to adjust the number of unlicensed contemporaries appearing in the probate accounts. Thus the strength of the total contingent serving the dying may be established.

The mean post-licensing lifespan for licensed practitioners for whom there are records of death and records of their activity recorded in the probate accounts is 24.2 years, to which the two years pre-licensing service needs to be added. The mean of the period between first appearance in a probate account and death is 18.3 years (making no adjustment for probate account dates), and thus it may be supposed that this group began serving the dying 7.7 years before the date of the probate account in which they are first mentioned. The period of 18.3 years compares with a mean of 14.4 years for unlicensed personnel mentioned in the probate accounts for whom there is a record of death. Whether unlicensed practitioners lived as long as licentiates it is not possible to say, but if it is assumed that they attended the seriously ill and dying for a period comparable to the average licentiate, then it follows that the average named practitioner had been active for about ten years before the first time he appears in a probate account. This allows us to account for the number of practitioners to whom there is certain reference and their likely numbers in any given year, where their first recorded reference in a probate account is between [16XX – 14] and [16XX + 10] inclusive (presuming a total medical lifespan of twenty-five years).

The above is, of course, inadequate as a total estimation of the numbers of unlicensed practitioners attending the dying. It is heavily dependent on the numbers of extant accounts: years with many accounts are likely to yield more names of unlicensed practitioners. Also, the propensity to record names itself may have changed. A correction factor therefore needs to be applied to these figures. The only correction which can be directly determined with a degree of justification is the proportion of practitioners who are known to have received a licence but who are not mentioned in any probate accounts. In theory, assuming that the names of unlicensed practitioners were recorded in the probate accounts as frequently as those of licentiates, the number of unlicensed practitioners may be adjusted proportionately. With these figures it is possible to estimate the total for the diocese of all sorts of medical practitioners who might be named in these accounts.

It is possible to run a partial check on these figures. If unlicensed and licensed practitioners are regarded as aspects of total practitioner employment at any given time, then by assessing the proportion of total practitioner employment undertaken by licensed and unlicensed practitioners (as recorded in the accounts) then the total number of practitioners may be extrapolated from the number of licentiates active at any given time. The resulting practitioner numbers, although less precise, are within 5 per cent of the results tabulated, the exception being the figures for 1710 (for which comparatively few probate accounts are extant).[4] Both methods indicate an almost identical number of practitioners in East Kent in the periods 1620–40 and 1670–1710, around the 190–5 mark. If the population of East Kent was increasing in the later part of the century, this is tantamount to a slight

---

4   Ibid. i. 159.

Table 28
Unlicensed practitioners in East Kent

Date	'Licensed' practitioners, incl. pre-licensed (A)	'Licensed' practitioners named in probate accounts (B)	Correction factor (A/B)	Unlicensed practitioners active	Total unlicensed practitioners (multiplied by A/B)
1620	87	30	2.9	31	90
1630	83	34	2.4	36	86
1640	85	34	2.5	37	92
1650	[data n/a]	–	–	–	–
1660	[data n/a]	38	–	–	–
1670	[98]	44	2.2	50	[110]
1680	[117]	56	2.1	58	[122]
1690	54	29	1.9	52	99
1700	58	29	2.0	31	62
1710	68	25	2.7	29	78

decline in practitioner: patient ratios, from about 191:75,000 (1:390) in 1620–40 to about 195:80,000 (1:410) in 1670–1710.[5]

Unfortunately it is not possible to replicate such methods of estimating practitioner numbers for any other county in this study. The records of practitioners are sparse or incomplete, and the probate accounts in other jurisdictions mention so few practitioners by name that it would be unwise to draw conclusions. Diocesan licences granted in Devon and Cornwall seem very slightly to have increased in numbers over the period, but in relation to the population the ratio of licentiates probably slightly declined. Also, of course, licentiates were proportionately much more thinly scattered than in East Kent. Unfortunately there are no probate account records of unlicensed activity in Devon and Cornwall. There are freemen figures for Exeter, and these do show a significant increase in the numbers of medical practitioners becoming freemen. For example, using the post-freedom lifespan of twenty-six years established for Canterbury, it is likely that in 1620 there were nine apothecaries and nine 'barbers'; whereas in 1691 it is likely that there were twenty-five apothecaries, two druggists, twenty-one 'barbers' and a 'chirurgeon' among the freemen.[6] However, it is not clear whether this increase in

---

[5] The increased population is based on Chalklin's estimates for Kent as a whole. His figures suggest that Kent grew from about 130,000 in 1600 to about 150,000 in 1676: *Seventeenth-century Kent*, 27.

[6] *Exeter freemen, 1266–1967*, ed. M. M. Rowe and A. M. Jackson (Devon and Cornwall Record Society e.s. i, 1973), 110–21.

Table 29
Total numbers of practitioners in East Kent

Date	'Licensed' practitioners, incl. pre-licensed	Canterbury freemen (from table 27)	Unlicensed/ non-freemen practitioners (from table 28)	Total practitioners
1620	87	15	90	192
1630	83	16	86	185
1640	85	19	92	196
1620–40	85	17	89	191
1650	[data n/a]	16	–	–
1660	[data n/a]	11	–	–
1670	[98]	13	[110]	[221]
1680	[117]	21	122	[260]
1690	54	24	99	177
1700	58	27	62	147
1710	68	25	78	171
1670–1710	79	22	94	195

numbers was also an increase or decrease in practitioner: population ratios for the region generally.

The only means of even remotely comparing numbers of practitioners in the various regions is through an assessment of diocesan licentiate: population ratios. By checking how many named practitioners in the probate accounts for each county were diocesan licentiates, total practitioner: population ratios may be estimated for that county at that time. Calculating the ratios for East Kent in this way suggests 1:384 in 1620 and 1:390 in 1690. In Wiltshire the twenty-six-year period 1664–89 (coinciding with the approximate length of the average East Kent practitioner's careerspan) may be evaluated. During this time nineteen diocesan licences were granted to practitioners to operate within Wiltshire, or men from Wiltshire were licensed to operate throughout the diocese. In this same period twenty-five individual practitioners were named in the probate accounts of whom only three were licensed by the diocese. On the basis of these small figures a total practitioner: population ratio might tentatively be estimated at 19: (120,000 x 3/25) = 1:760. This goes some way to explaining why, in Wiltshire, medical assistance to the dying remained exclusively an urban and high-status choice even in the later seventeenth century. There were only half as many practitioners per head of the population, and the Wiltshire population itself was far more spread out, the county being much less-densely settled.

No other licensing and probate accounts series is sufficiently complete to warrant a similar estimate. The nearest is the twenty-four years of licensing for West Sussex (1661–84), during which period twenty diocesan licences were granted for residents in an archdeaconry of about 50,000. The proportion of practitioners named in the Chichester probate accounts who were licensed was 5/19. If it is asssumed that these twenty practitioners in twenty-four years is the equivalent of twenty-two in twenty-six years, a ratio of $22:(50,000 \times 5/19) = 1:600$ may be estimated. An intermediary ratio of practitioners to population would explain why some features in West Sussex do compare with East Kent while others – the rural disadvantage, for example – do not.

Practitioner distribution

The important point to emerge from these figures is that there is no indication of an increase in practitioner numbers in East Kent at all, let alone one commensurate with the very substantial increase in the use of medicine by the dying over the seventeenth century. It follows that the massive increases in the medicalisation of serious illnesses and fatal cases was not merely a symptom of the whole of society – young and old, slightly unwell and seriously ill – becoming more medicalised. The tendency to seek medical assistance for dealing with a broken limb or arthritis, for example, could not have increased by 400/500 per cent without a very large increase in practitioner numbers. Nevertheless, even though the medicalisation that is being measured was specifically on behalf of the seriously ill, it is necessary to ask how it could happen. How could the East Kent practitioners serve so many more seriously ill people throughout the whole diocese if their total numbers were not increasing?

Part of the answer to this question lies in understanding that most illnesses and ailments do not require medical attention. Even today the majority of injuries and slight sicknesses are dealt with in the home. Ronald Sawyer cites a modern study which suggests that 93 per cent of ailments and illnesses are dealt with domestically.[7] It follows that for a society to become 'medicalised' in a modern sense, only the most serious 7 per cent of ailments require expert medical help. The question is thus one of how an unenlarged body of practitioners could go from satisfying this 7 per cent requirement in 5 per cent of the population to satisfying it in the majority within two generations. It is possible that they dealt more regularly with the serious cases by dealing less regularly with the minor ones, leaving these to womenfolk and the readers of self-help books. Certainly licensed physicians after 1660 would not have been consulted regularly on relatively minor matters such as astrology and the occult (as Simon Forman was in the first decade of the century). In this way the more serious, dedicated medical practitioners could give more of their time to the seriously ill. This in turn points to a second part of

---

7   Sawyer, 'Patients, healers', 178.

Table 30
East Kent practitioners living outside towns

	No. with known residence	No. resident >1 mile from a medical town	No. in probate accts with known residence	No. in probate accts resident >1 mile from town
1590–1619	129	28 (22%)	66	9 (14%)
1620–49	130	27 (21%)	65	12 (18%)
1660–89	226	60 (27%)	119	23 (19%)
1690–1719	110	42 (38%)	38	12 (32%)

the answer: changes in the nature of medical assistance itself. As distant, lengthy consultations involving astrological prediction and urine-inspection gave way to chemical medicines, involving little more than consultation and a prescription, then it is clear how the physicians of Kent could cope with a greatly increased workload.

A third part of the answer has to do with the rural aspect of the increase in medical assistance. As hinted at in a previous chapter medical practitioners increasingly settled in rural areas in the later seventeenth century, thereby increasing their availability in the region through greater geographic distribution. Two regions particularly noted as having few practitioners in the early years of the seventeenth century – Thanet and Lydd – were served by several practitioners by the end of the century, and the number of individuals benefiting from those services went up very substantially in those areas. The increase in the numbers of rural practitioners may be measured in several ways, for instance the proportions resident outside medical towns who served the dying. Although, unfortunately, data on places of residence for all practitioners are not available, the figures provided in table 30 seem unambiguous.

The figures in the first two columns are tentative, for in most cases the parish of residence has to be presumed to be the parish used in the licence. This is usually the home parish, or parish of training, and there are undoubtedly cases where the practitioner later moved. For this reason, the next two columns must be considered a more accurate view. However, even these more reliable numbers do not reveal the whole extent of medical rustification. When the places of residence of locatable licentiates are examined, it is clear that not only were more practitioners living away from medical towns, they were also living further away from medical towns (*see* table table 31).

To put these figures into context, the mean distance of all parishes from 'medical towns' in East Kent was 3.2 miles (in Sussex 3.6 and Berkshire 3.9 miles). Thus, even though there were no more practitioners in the region in 1680–1700 than in the first half of the century, they were living in greater proximity to the rural inhabitants. This suggests not just an easier journey to

Table 31
Average distances of diocesan-licensed practitioners' home towns from medical towns in East Kent

	'Physic'		'Surgery'		Phys. & Surg.	
	Avg dist.	No.	Avg dist.	No.	Avg dist.	No.
1590–1619	0.7	18	1.5	58	0	1
1620–49	1.0	18	1.1	40	0	1
1660–89	1.6	24	1.8	93	0.4	8
1690–1719	2.2	4	2.5	51	2.6	7

get medical help or advice, but a stronger relationship between rural parish communities and medical practitioners, and probably a greater familiarity with both the practitioner and the espoused advantages of medical assistance. By 1700, in East Kent at least, a relationship of proximity existed between a licensed practitioner and a community comparable to that of a general practitioner throughout the country in the next century, and comparable to the early seventeenth-century rural Buckinghamshire practice of Richard Napier, discussed by Ronald Sawyer.[8]

In the West Country it is clear that similar relationships were developing between communities and practitioners at this time. Although there were many fewer licentiates, the large numbers of signatures on 'petitions' for practitioners to obtain licences were effectively attempts by communities – usually small towns – to recognise a local practitioner officially and to disenfranchise his medical rivals.[9] Local authorities could prevent their community from being visited by itinerant quacks, or, if quacks did visit, the authorities could deprive them of the right legally to practise without jeopardising their established medical service. What is particularly interesting is that this appears to have happened in large towns as well as in the small ones. The mayor of Plymouth headed the list of signatories on one such petition in 1715, and the mayor of Okehampton submitted one in 1665. In these towns the emphasis may well have been on favouring particularly well-connected practitioners or those who were acting on behalf of the poor of the town. A number of petitions stress the numbers of poor people cured, and a town's action in effectively appointing its principal physician or surgeon helped not only to secure the services of a trusted practitioner but also established an exclusive market for his services at the same time. If closer ties were being made between communities and practitioners in towns as well as rural parishes, this might explain why practitioners were inclined to settle in further-flung areas. It was not just in response to demand for their

8   Ibid. 194–6.
9   Mortimer, 'Diocesan licensing', 66.

services but in reaction to increased difficulties in finding a footing within the towns.

In East Kent it seems that a similar system was at work. Two 1661 petitions for Maidstone practitioners were signed by at least twenty substantial local men. Late seventeenth-century petitions with seven or more signatures are to be found for Ashford, Brabourne, Canterbury, Challock, Charing, Cranbrook, Dover (2), Egerton, Elham (2), Goudhurst (2), Marden, Pankhurst, Sittingbourne (4), Smeeth and Warden.[10] As in Devon and Cornwall, these petitions form the minority of types of extant supporting documentation for licence applications. In most cases it appears that the testimony of the more influential established medical practitioners was the preferred (and in Devon and Cornwall at least, more successful) method of obtaining a licence. But the frequent survival of evidence of community approval in both dioceses, for both small towns and large ones, suggests that in the far south-east as in the far south-west, the recruitment and retention of medical practitioners mattered greatly to the community, to the extent that many communities in East Kent seem to have made efforts to attract a licensed practitioner to act locally.

If licentiates were spreading out across rural areas of East Kent, and Canterbury freemen practitioners were town-based (with the exceptions of those notable country physicians like Robert Pemell, who received their freedoms as an honour), what can be said about the regional distribution of the remainder, the unlicensed? These are a harder group to assess, since comparatively fewer home towns are known; but for the most part it appears that they remained town-based.

In contrast to the licentiates, as far as can be established unlicensed practitioners seem only very slowly to have shifted away from towns to practise in rural areas. No practitioner working outside a town is ever described as an apothecary. The two payments noted in the probate accounts to identified church ministers for medical assistance are for the earlier periods. Since table 32 probably includes some practitioners with official credentials who do not happen to have received a licence from the diocese or archbishop, or the freedom of the City of Canterbury – some medical degree-holders, for example – it is a reasonable postulation that those with recognised qualifications (mostly licentiates) found it easier to gain acceptance in rural communities. Practitioner numbers might have been falling slightly in the late seventeenth century, but the distribution of licentiates seems to have been more even. Combined with possible changes in the nature of medical assistance, it would appear that greater rural dissemination allowed an unchanging number of practitioners to satisfy the greatly increased medical demands of a larger proportion of dying people.

10 Wellcome Trust Library, MS 5343.

Table 32
Unlicensed practitioners in East Kent in relation to the nearest medical town

Occupational description	1590–1619 Avg dist.	No.	1620–49 Avg dist.	No.	1660–89 Avg dist.	No.	1690–1719 Avg dist.	No.
Apothecary	0.0	4	0.0	7	0.0	8	0.0	2
Barber/ B-surgeon	0.0	1	0.0	2	4.5	2	–	0
Church minister	4.0	1	3.0	1	–	0	–	0
Physician (incl. 'Dr')	0.7	11	0.2	13	0.6	20	0.0	4
Physician &/or Surgeon	–	0	0.0	1	0.0	3	2.5	2
Surgeon	1.1	8	2.6	6	1.3	25	2.1	7
Uncertain	0.5	5	2.0	8	1.7	3	0.0	2
Totals	0.8	30	1.0	38	1.0	61	1.1	17

Practitioner identities

Turning from gross numbers of medical practitioners, it is now necessary to analyse the detailed make-up of the medical personnel that we have been trying to enumerate and locate. This is not just a matter of how many apothecaries and surgeons were around at a given time but the nature of their practices, that is to say, what was a surgeon in 1620 as opposed to 1690? Were all apothecaries performing similar roles? Was there a potential for conflict between surgeons and physicians in 1690 which previously had not existed?

In answering such questions consideration may be given to a breakdown of identified practitioners licensed or granted the freedom of Canterbury between 1590 and 1719, or first recorded in a probate account or other source between those dates.

Table 33 confirms something most medical historians have long understood: occupational epithets owed as much to the context in which they were written down as the boundaries of the occupations (real or imagined) to which they related. The licensing authorities, constrained by the terms of the early sixteenth-century legislation, operated within a rigid legal framework in which only the terms 'surgery', 'medicine' (or 'physic') and 'midwifery' were meaningful. This rigidity began to give way in the decades around 1700 as licences to practise both medicine and surgery were more frequently granted in the dioceses of Canterbury and Exeter (to name just two).[11] It was not until the 1730s that Exeter began to award licences for surgery and

---

[11] See Mortimer, 'Diocesan licensing', 52.

Table 33
Practitioner descriptions according to source and representation in probate accounts

Style	Dioc. Lics	Arch. Lics	Freemen	Others	Total named in accounts, 1590–1719
'Apothecary'	–	–	43	24	40
'Barber-surgeon'	–	–	34	5	5
[Church minister]	–	–	–	2	2
'Dr' or 'Physician'	71	18	5	95	138
'Physician & surgeon'	15	14	–	10	15
'Surgeon'	255	8	22	70	152
[Uncertain]	–	4	–	70	65
Total	341	44	104	276	417

Note: Some of the apothecaries and surgeons are described interchangeably in some accounts.

pharmacy, and similarly no licence granted by the diocese of Canterbury made reference to pharmacy or strayed from the legal remit before 1730. In this sense a 'surgeon', as defined by a diocesan licence, was different from a freeman 'surgeon': a practitioner licensed by the diocese to perform surgery might be called an apothecary or a physician by the world at large. Similarly a townsman licensed by the diocese to practise 'medicine' need not necessarily have been regarded purely as a physician by the majority of his clientele, some of whom might have regarded him as an apothecary. Walter Southwell of Canterbury was described as an apothecary in the register of Canterbury freemen, and was usually described as an apothecary in the various probate accounts which mention him, but he also held a diocesan licence to practice surgery. Similarly Peter Annott of Canterbury, who received an archiepiscopal licence for 'physic and surgery' in 1594, was described in the probate accounts relating to him as either a 'physician' or 'surgeon' but not both. Alexander Devison, licensed to perform surgery, was sometimes described as a surgeon and sometimes as a physician in the probate accounts. William Fox likewise was licensed as a 'surgeon', and was indeed described as 'surgeon' in at least three accounts, but he was also described as 'barber-surgeon' and 'physician' in others. The occupational descriptions associated with the arts to which licences related did not necessarily restrict individuals to an occupational creed or medical philosophy. Rather it would appear that licences represented a legal status – and perhaps a degree of social status and proficiency – more than a professional designation.

Those who did not hold licences were even more likely to be given a variety of occupational descriptors by accountants. William Allen, described as a surgeon in his probate inventory, was called an apothecary in one of the three accounts relating to his services. George Baily, an apothecary (according to his own probate account), was described as a physician in the records relating to his activities. Claude Clare or Clear (d.1692) of Hythe was described as a physician in 1684, as a doctor in 1685 and 1691, and as a surgeon in 1691. John Boughton (d.1692) of Elham, described as a surgeon in his probate inventory, was referred to as a chirurgion in the years 1670, 1688 and 1691 but as a physician in accounts dated 1673, 1674, 1675, 1676, 1680 and 1682. Most of the references to this man describe him providing physic and travelling to the patient and giving advice about the medicines he prescribed, so it is not surprising to find him also described as a doctor in two accounts. There are dozens of similar examples: inconsistency of nomenclature was almost as common as consistency. Freemen apothecaries were frequently described as physicians; and, like licensed physicians, they might also be described as surgeons in the context of performing surgery. Physicians and licensed surgeons supposed by accountants to be 'physicians' were frequently accorded the pretitle 'Doctor' whether or not they held a degree, especially in the later seventeenth century. Occupational descriptions of practitioners refer to general or specific functions, roles or specialisms, not integral occupations. There are a few exceptions to the rule of variable nomenclature – no person described as an apothecary can be associated with any place of residence other than one of the designated 'medical towns' – but even so the majority of seventeenth-century provincial practitioners cannot be regarded as belonging to distinct occupations. The account of Susan Omer explicitly describes the same distillation being made by an 'apothecary' and a 'physician', thus further blurring the medical roles.[12] Someone who sold drugs from a shop might be termed an apothecary, but if he travelled to a man's house to cut off his leg, he might be termed a surgeon; and if he advised the man in his melancholy state after the amputation, he might be termed a physician. If this sequence of events had taken place in the latter half of the seventeenth century, the patient might well have referred to him in conversation as 'the doctor'.

The upshot of this is that the apothecary, the surgeon and the physician cannot be regarded as involved in distinct occupations with clearly and exclusively defined responsibilities. Contemporaries did not always know the occupational identity of a practitioner, or even whether the practitioner himself had adopted a single occupational identity, even though he may have had his own preferred designation. Several examples may be noted of named practitioners being described as 'a phisition or chirurgion'.[13] These, like the examples of practitioners being accorded separate occupational

---

[12] PRC 2/31/53.
[13] Three such being Edward Anderson of Sandwich, Mr Grosham, and Thomas Day of Dover: Mortimer, 'Directory'.

identities by separate accountants, demonstrate that occupational identities were conflated in general by society and by the clients who employed them.

On this point, it is worth remarking that historians have not hitherto had access to large numbers of records of doubtful practitioner nomenclature, only records of occupational identities in specific and limited contexts. Thus the traditional 'tripartite hierarchy' expressed by contemporaries has been maintained by many writers – often with a note of caution – simply because they had no evidence as to how strong or weak this concept was. For example, Ronald Sawyer could write that 'barbers [i.e. barber-surgeons] gained their identity through a guild structure'; yet from the evidence presented here it is clear that practitioner identities were much more amorphous than the systematic assignment of names in gild registers. Margaret Pelling has demonstrated that practitioners themselves were conscious of different identities while yet being members of a single barbers' company.[14] The probate accounts show very clearly that the blurring of identities extended throughout the community. In the diocese of Canterbury many physicians were so described by their non-medical contemporaries on account of their dispensing physic, not because of an exclusive identity at the head of a tripartite hierarchy. Although the sense in which the physician was the head of such a hierarchy may have had relevance in London, where the College of Physicians asserted its rights, to equate this with the situation in the provinces is like comparing the monarch and House of Lords with the mayor and aldermen of a provincial town.

The lack of strict identities casts doubt on the idea that it was only in small towns that practitioners' services overlapped.[15] William Fox, a licensed surgeon also described as a physician and a barber-surgeon, lived in Canterbury. Thomas Wildes, an apothecary licensed to practise surgery, lived in Dover. John Woolshaffen of Canterbury, several times described as 'Dr Woolshaffen', was a freeman apothecary licensed to perform surgery. So too was Walter Southwell. William Sandford was a freeman apothecary licensed to practise medicine. At least fifteen Canterbury freemen were also licentiates. Some licentiates were also degree-holders, and some practitioners had multiple 'qualifications': John Bale and Alexander Capell, both of Canterbury, each had a diocesan licence, an archiepiscopal licence and a medical degree. While some practitioners restricted themselves to just one medical function – for example, running an apothecary's shop – and thus were never accorded a second occupational identity in their whole career, many others had more than one string to their bow. Furthermore, as Margaret Pelling has pointed out, these were not always medical occupations.[16] Renting property was a common parallel income stream for medical practitioners (as it

14 Sawyer, 'Patients, healers', 100; M. Pelling, *The common lot*, London 1998, 208–9.
15 R. Porter, 'The patient in England, c. 1660–1800', in A. Wear (ed.), *Medicine in society*, Cambridge 1992, 92–3.
16 Pelling, *Common lot*, 222–5.

71

was for much of the affluent population); but lending money, ship-owning and funeral assistance were also part-time occupations for practitioners in East Kent.[17] In one case an individual was paid for giving the son of the deceased music lessons in addition to 'looking after' his diseased leg.[18] When these versatile practitioners were employed on behalf of the dying, it was the medical service for which they had been paid which mattered to the dead patient's next of kin (the authors of most of these accounts), and it was in the context of the service rendered to their late father, husband, brother, sister or mother that the creator of an account assigned an identity to the practitioner. Hence a specific service was often described as being performed by 'a phisition or a chirurgion'.

It is also important not to underestimate the extent to which the social definitions of medical designations changed over time. The key descriptors used for both the higher status groups and the lower status groups in East Kent vary considerably from one generation to the next. For both groups the most commonly used epithet was 'surgeon' in accounts dated 1570–1619, but it was 'physician' in the period 1620–49.[19] After the Restoration the term 'doctor' became as widely used as 'physician' (even more so for the higher status group), and in both groups apothecaries and surgeons were comparatively rarely mentioned as such. In the last period, 1690–1719, the term 'doctor' was by far the most commonly used in respect of both groups.

Such shifting preferences appear in respect of geographical location too. In the period 1660–89 rural high-status accountants used the description 'physician' slightly more often than 'doctor' but their urban counterparts used the term 'doctor' much more commonly than 'physician'. Similarly amongst those of lesser status there was a three times greater use made of the description 'apothecary' by those in towns in the period 1620–89 than those of similar status in rural areas (for whom 'physician' was a more frequently applied term). This might indicate that townsmen were buying more medicines from pharmaceutical tradesmen than rural inhabitants, but it might

---

[17] For examples of practitioners renting property see especially PRC 19/6/70, which has an entry 'paid more to the said Mr Thomas Knowler for looking after and administering phisick to her the said deceased and Richard Crofts her late husband'. The previous entry includes payments to Mr Thomas Knowler and brokers for rent £26, and another to Mr T Knowler £10 for rent. The following entries may also be considered with regard to rent: 'To him [Mr Day, surgeon] more due by the said deceased for rent due by the deceased and for attendance on her in her sicknes £4': PRC 19/3/55; 'To Mr Henry Tritton of Ashford barber, for rent': PRC 2/31/40; 'Paid to Mr Avery Hills [a freeman apothecary of Canterbury] for rent due unto him by the said deceased at his death £7 4s': PRC 20/13/1. The account of Elnathan Hannam, surgeon, records that he owned parts of 2 vessels lost at sea: PRC 20/12/306. Mr Joseph Colfe of Canterbury, alderman and apothecary/physician, was owed 20s. for beer: PRC 2/27/161. Most apothecaries also stocked Naples Biscuit etc for funerals; some also provided coffins.

[18] The entry reads 'paid to Mr Patino ... for looking after Peter Duflo [son of the deceased] legg and teaching him to sing, 43s 2d': PRC 19/5/53 (1697).

[19] Mortimer, 'Medical assistance', ii. 61–2.

equally indicate that 'apothecary' was merely the term more commonly used in towns, and that rural folk called these practitioners 'physicians'. In the late sixteenth century there was a greater use made of the description 'surgeon' by those of lower status in towns than in the country (52 per cent compared to 33 per cent of those with descriptions supplied), but this does not necessarily indicate that surgery was more frequently performed, for a 'physician' or 'doctor' might carry out surgical operations more frequently in the country. All that is certain is that contemporary nomenclature was subject to a wide range of local, social and occupational influences; and that the terms used reflected the service paid for on behalf of the deceased. This is subject to the clarification that the very terms applied changed their meaning, or were at some times and in some places more readily used by the accountant and the court clerk than at other times and in other places.

As a result, when examining medical assistance to the dying, it is not possible to choose whether to approach the subject from the point of view of practitioners or their services. The provision of 'physic' cannot be sepa-rated from the roles of the 'physician', the 'apothecary' or the 'surgeon', and nor can 'medicines' be treated as distinct from 'physic' or 'apothecary stuff' or 'ointments'. The role of 'physicians' in the late sixteenth century cannot be examined with the presumption that this group represents the profes-sional antecedents of 'physicians' in the late seventeenth. The same goes for doctors and surgeons. The only way systematically to proceed is to examine the language used in context: the words with which accountants and clerks described services rendered to the dying, and the nomenclature of the prac-titioners who performed those services at various times.

Medical services

'Physic'

By far the most commonly described medical service to the dying mentioned in the probate accounts was the provision of 'physic'. In many cases – probably most cases – this may be taken to mean the provision or purchase of medic-inal substances, but often the reference was a general one, which in some instances included medical advice and/or surgical assistance, and in others may have referred only to medical advice or surgery. Contemporary defini-tions of 'physic' accentuate this catch-all definition: Blount's *Glossographia* (2nd edn, 1661) equates 'physick' with 'medicine' and describes it as being 'of five kinds: 1. *Pharmaceutic*, cureth diseases by application of medicaments. 2. *Chirurgic*, by incision or cauterizing. 3. *Diætetic*, by diet. 4. *Nosognomonick* discerns diseases. 5. *Boethetic* removes them.'[20] Edward Phillips described 'physick' in his *New world of English words* (1657) as 'naturall philosophy:

---

[20] T. Blount, *Glossographia*, 2nd edn, London 1661.

also the art of curing by medicines'.[21] Along the same lines, in his *English dictionary* three decades later, Elisha Coles differentiated between '*Physicks*: Natural Philosophy' and '*Physick*: medicine'.[22] In the *Physicall dictionary*, first published in the same year as Phillips's work, the term is not described at all but rather is that by which the whole field of medicine may be known, the same title being given to Stephen Blancard's work of 1684.[23]

Such an all-encompassing definition is evidenced throughout the probate accounts. That it could mean medical substances administered by a physician is frequently made clear in such lines as 'paid to Mr Pistoll phisition ... for phisick by him administred' and 'paid to Mr Cleere Apothecary ... for phisicke by him administred to the said deceased' both of which are from accounts dated 1674.[24] Such entries are very common in respect of both 'apothecaries' and 'physicians'. That men described as 'surgeons' and 'barber-surgeons' also might equally dispense 'physic' is not in doubt.[25] Accounts such as that of Thomas Godfrey, which includes the entry 'paid vnto Mr Thomas Annott of the same [Faversham] Chirurgion for phisick or chirurgery minis-tred by him to the said deceased in the tyme of the sicknes whereof he dyed' raise the question of whether 'physic' could also relate to a surgical activity.[26] And of course the word 'physic' could be used in respect of an occupational description, as shown in two adjacent accounts dated 1636: 'paid and laid out to Mr Thomas Lennard Doctor of Phisick for his paines and attend-ance in the office of a phisitian vpon the said deceased testator' and 'paid to Mr John Greenleafe of the Cittie of Canterbury phisition & apothecary for phisicall thinges advice & attendance on the said deceased testator'.[27] Obviously no generalisations about the nature of services rendered can be made on the strength of payments for 'physic', nor about the occupation of the person supplying such a service.

One significant opportunity for the historian lies in this very vagueness of medical description: the many payments for 'physic' may be used to establish a basic comparative estimate of the costs as provided by variously described practitioners to different status groups. Since the term 'physic' was used so frequently and with regard to patients of all status groups across the whole period, by examining those payments which are exclusively single payments

[21] E. Phillips, *A new world of English words*, 1st edn, London 1657.

[22] E. Coles, *An English dictionary*, 2nd edn, London 1685.

[23] Anon., *A physicall dictionary*, London 1657; S. Blancard, *A physical dictionary; in which all the terms relating either to anatomy, chirugery, pharmacy, or chymistry, are very accurately explain'd*, London 1684.

[24] PRC 2/36/2–3. The two accounts are archivally adjacent.

[25] More than sixty Kent accounts record payments to surgeons for 'physic'. See Mortimer, 'Medical assistance', ii. 214 (entry under John Fox, 1692), which reads 'paid to John Fox, surgeon for Phisick'.

[26] PRC 2/21/37.

[27] PRC 2/33/100.

Table 34
Average sums paid for 'physic'

	East Kent		West Sussex, Berkshire and Wiltshire	
	Status A, B, R	Status C, D, S	Status A, B, R	Status C, D, S
1570–1619	18.1	10.1	17.1	12.3
1620–49	30.2	15.4	26.4	21.4
1660–89	31.5	18.8	35.5	21.7
1690–1719	38.4	20.5	–	–

Note: All sums expressed in shillings.

Figure 9
Average sums paid for 'physic' in East Kent

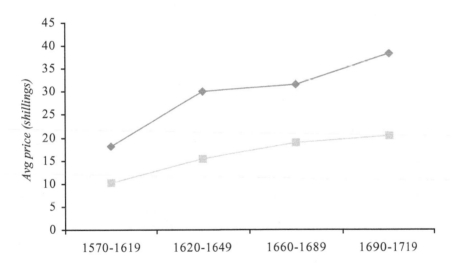

for 'physic', and averaging the amounts recorded, a rough price index of 'physic' provided to the seriously ill and dying may be obtained.[28]

Using this approach the charges for 'physic' in East Kent may be compared with those in the other counties for which accounts are extant, according to status groups. Although numbers of payments purely for 'physic' are comparatively few in number outside Kent, the general trends in East Kent are very similar to those which may be noted in central southern England.

---

28 Mortimer, 'Medical assistance', ii. 63–6.

Medicines, ointments and drugs

It is with specific forms of 'physic' that the subject of what services were being obtained by the dying and who was supplying them can be more confidently approached. Still it is not a precise area of study. There are economic issues to consider as well as problems of definition. On the economic side it is rarely possible to distinguish between 'medicines' which formed the whole service purchased, and medicines which formed only a part of a service, for example ointments applied in addition to surgery. In relation to 'doctors' this extends to payments for 'physic and advice' which almost certainly relates to both medicines and consultation. With regard to problems of definition, 'medicines' may include ointments, which were traditionally external and thus aspects of surgery, as well as internal medicines (which were an aspect of a physician's art). Even more important, a number of purchases of 'medicines' were undoubtedly confused with 'necessaries', being medicinal in the opinion of one accountant and merely 'necessary' in another's view.

To illustrate this problem and examine its impact, it is worth considering the middle ground between 'necessaries' and 'medicines'. The East Kent accounts record more than 200 instances of 'necessaries' or essential provisions being purchased for the deceased in his or her last days. These may be described simply in general terms, such as 'to Mr Mullenexe ... for necessary thinges <fetched> in the time of his last sicknes'[29] or in a more precise manner, such as 'for sugar, cloves a white loaf and a pott of beere (7d) and a pound of candles (5d), a neck of mutton (8d), a brest of mutton (9d), for bred (5d), great candles (2d), 5 potts of beere and 4 loves [loaves] (9d), more bread (3d)',[30] or in a semi-specific way, for example 'paid for spyces and other necessaryes ffor the said testator in the tyme of his sickenes'[31] or 'paid for physick and other necessaryes for the said William Norington in the tyme of his sickenes'.[32] The first three of these four examples may be construed simply as 'necessary' in that they were the essential provisions to sustain the bed-ridden or dying patient. On the other hand, 'necessary' referred to spices, alcohol and meat – especially mutton – obtained as part of the special or ritual treatment of the sick. In this sense, although a leg of mutton was not something obtained from a medical practitioner, it might have been obtained with a remedial or palliative purpose in mind. This also applies to the quantities of beer, aquavite and wine purchased during the time of sickness, for example 'paid for wine for him in his sicknes'[33] or 'for wine and several necessaries had for the said deceased in the time of the sickness he

29 PRC 2/25/62.
30 PRC 20/3/318.
31 PRC 2/4/511.
32 PRC 2/7/263.
33 PRC 1/17/69.

died of, the particulars whereof this accomptant is ready to produce'.[34] A remedial function is even more overtly demonstrated in the payments for broths, apparently cooked especially for the ill person, which are evidenced in such payments as 'paid for a quarte of muskaden, a quarte of sacke, for a cocke, and ... for fruite for broathes and for milke in the time of the sicknes whereof she died'[35] and 'payd for a necke of mutton and fruite to make the sayd deceaseds broath whilest he liued'.[36] In this way it may be seen that, while normal provision was 'necessary', so too were remedial provisions, which included some home-spun medicinal processes, from broths to spiced food, roots, fruit, and other herbal and medicinal substances obtained from an apothecary.

Having stressed the blurred lines between ordinary and extraordinary provision which may lie behind the wording used in these accounts, it has to be admitted that the only sensible way of considering the evidence relating to medicines is to interpret the words used literally, i.e. to exclude all references such as 'paid and laid out for watch candles, liquorish and figs for the said deceased in the time of his visitation'[37] in favour of those which explicitly mention 'medicines', or 'ointments'. The East Kent accounts include about 240 direct references to the purchase or administration of some form of 'medicines' or medical substance, not including references to 'physic' but including payments for medicines in conjunction with physical advice or surgery. This is sufficient for certain suggestions to be advanced about the provision of medicines in East Kent (*see* table 35).

The prices paid for medicines followed a significant upward trend until the Restoration period, comparable to that noted for physic generally and well in excess of what might have been expected based on general price indexes derived from probate inventories.[38] What is interesting about the figures presented in table 35 is that, while apothecaries remained the dominant traders for the supply of medicines, their financial benefit from the trade in substances was comparatively slight by comparison with that achieved by some surgeons in the late sixteenth and early seventeenth centuries. At the period when 'surgeon' was the epithet most commonly applied to medical practitioners serving the dying, there are some large payments to them for medicines. In later years, when 'doctor' and 'physician' had become the descriptors of choice, men so described were able to charge higher fees. Unfortunately there are too few examples to be certain, but it is a distinct possibility that there is a correlation between the most popular term used to describe practitioners and the ability of practitioners so described to charge

---

34 Ibid.
35 PRC 2/32/129.
36 PRC 2/26/91.
37 PRC 1/4/66.
38 See Overton, 'Prices from inventories', 140.

Table 35
East Kent payments for medical substances in relation to practitioner designation

	1570–1619		1620–49		1660–89		1690–1719	
	No.	Avg price	No.	Avg price	No.	Avg price	No.	Avg price
Apothecary	25	9.6	29	24.9	26	51.0	13	37.5
Doctor	2	6.25	1	14.0	4	33.1	2	17.5
Physician	0	-	13	13.4	16	47.2	3	62.1
Surgeon	6	46.3	7	105.5	5	14.7	6	21.1
Not stated	19	11.1	14	21.8	11	36.9	16	45.1
Totals	52	14.3	64	30.5	62	43.4	40	38.9

Note: Average (mean) prices are in shillings.

high fees, with the obvious implication for the occupational identities with which practitioners wished to be associated.

Another feature of medicines reflected in the probate accounts is that they did not always require the attendance of an occupationally defined medical practitioner to administer them. As shown by entries such as 'paide more vnto the saide Goodwife Sweyton for pottecarie ware which she fetched for the said John Wheeller deceased in the time of his last sickness', remedies could be 'fetched', their applications presumably being known to a member or an acquaintance of the household.[39] The self-help medical books in circulation probably aided in the selection and production of remedies. In some instances – for instance, plague – the popular medicines were as well known as the disease.[40] In such cases all one could do was to obtain the requisite medicine from an appropriate vendor. 'Paid for aquavitae & other drinkes necessaries of phisick the which was fetched for the deceased in the tyme of the sicknes whereof he died & due & to be payd at his deathe' shows 'necessary' drinks being purchased.[41] At the other extreme, the purchase of some medicines required the full assistance of one or more suitable practitioners in person. This might take the traditional form of prescription by a physician and supply of medicines by an apothecary, as in a 1583 case which simply reads 'payde to the Apothecary for drugges prescribed by the phisitian'.[42] But such instances are rare. Much more common is the assistance of a practitioner in aiding or advising in the administration of drugs. Thus, for example, 'paid to Mr Hughes of Ashford appothecrie for medicines & his

[39] PRC 2/14/494.
[40] On the high level of knowledge about the plague displayed by Napier's rural patients see Sawyer, 'Patients, healers', 430–40.
[41] PRC 20/1/1.
[42] PRC 2/3/41.

travayling to minister & apply the same to the said deceased in the tyme of his sicknes'.[43] Often, if a doctor or physician were specifically involved in the administration of medicines, the role of the doctor was not solely that of prescription but of application or administration of the medicines obtained. As a result, the generally accepted working of the tripartite hierarchy – that 'the physician prescribed and the apothecary provided' – is less than half the story. Leaving aside the self-prescribing role of the patient, it would be more accurate to say that, in East Kent, the physician prescribed, an apothecary or the said physician provided, and either the providing apothecary, the said physician or the patient himself administered. When surgeons were involved, normally both the provision of medicine and its application remained wholly within their control. This feature of surgical medicine remained the case in East Kent throughout the period under study.[44]

So who was providing the bulk of the medicines in East Kent? On the face of it, the answer is those described as 'apothecaries'. However there is a problem in assuming this; 'medicines' was a word more frequently used in respect of apothecaries and 'physic' was more frequently used in respect of physicians. Thus there is a bias in the language itself. To lessen the effect of this, a limited number of payments for physic may be examined. If it is assumed that, where practitioners were paid for 'physic and advice', 'physic' was synonymous with 'medicines', the bias inherent against physicians may be reduced. Taking just the instances where there was a sole practitioner designation associated with either a payment for 'medicines' or 'physick and advice', the designations applied to those providing medicinal substances may be shown.

It appears that the designation 'apothecary' was less frequently applied to the providers of medicines after 1660 than before, and the designations 'physician' and 'doctor' more frequently applied. If it is correct to assume that 'apothecary' as a designation was exclusively associated with men running shops in medical towns in East Kent throughout the period, then these changes are what might have been expected. Medicines were more frequently being obtained from the increasing numbers of rural practitioners, who were never described in East Kent as apothecaries.

---

[43] PRC 2/13/312.

[44] Specific examples include 'paid to Thomas Day Chirurgion for Cordialls by him administred to the said deceased in the time aforesaid': PRC 20/13/52; 'To Richard Wineatts of Sandwich, chirurgion, for comings over to the deceased when he was shutt up and for cordialls he gave then unto the family': PRC 1/2/76; 'paide to Thomas Waterman of Plucklie chiurgion for debte due to him by the saide deceassed at his deathe for looking to the saide deceassed & applying medycines vnto him in the tyme of his Sicknes': PRC 2/7/371; 'paid vnto raphe watson the surgeon for letting the said Anthony goddard blode and for oyntmentes and his paynes in attending vpon the said Antony in the tyme of his sickenes': PRC 2/8/177; 'paid to Mr Hammon chirurgeon for his attendance on the said deceased in his last sickness whereof he died and for medicine administered by him to the said deceased': PRC 1/17/76.

Table 36
Designations of East Kent practitioners providing 'medicines' or 'physic and advice'

	1570–1649	1660–1719
Apothecary	55	39
Druggist	0	1
Doctor	18	28
Physician	24	35
Surgeon	15	13
Barber	1	0
Not stated	40	35
Total	153	151

Note: Excludes ambiguous cases, for example 'paid to the physician and apothecary for medicine/physic and advice'.

Table 37
Designations of East Kent practitioners providing 'advice'

	1570–1649	1660–1719
Apothecary	2	0
Doctor	24	42
Physician	28	25
Surgeon	5	4
Not stated	15	8
Total	74	79

Note: Excludes ambiguous cases.

Advice and practitioner attendance

All designations of practitioner gave advice. Whether they were technically permitted to do so by the College of Physicians or not, it is a well-recorded aspect of medical assistance to the dying. The word 'advice' itself is recorded in 172 instances in the East Kent accounts and twenty-five cases outside Kent. Some of these are ambiguous, such as 'paid to the doctor and apothecary for advice and medicines' (in which cases assumptions have to be made in order to determine who was doing what). But laying aside all such ambiguous payments it is possible to establish which practitioner designations were most frequently associated with 'advising' the dying.

In both time frames the vast majority of practitioners paid for giving advice were described either as 'physician' or 'doctor'; in the earlier period 'physician' being the more common term, this situation being reversed after 1660. The traditional view of the physician's role is strikingly supported.

The term 'advice', however, is not without its ambiguities. For a start there is a great difference between specific advice on the taking of medi-cines, and general advice about a patient's condition. The former relates to a process already decided upon, whereas the latter relates to consultation, perhaps prior to any decision-making. And consultation did not necessarily lead to medicines being taken; there are several probable cases of second or multiple opinions being called for. Nor was such advice necessarily remedial; in some cases it probably included information touching upon the period of life remaining in which the patient might set his affairs in order. With this in mind it cannot be stated on the basis of the figures given so far that most diagnoses were the work of physicians. A practitioner described as a 'surgeon' may also have acted in a diagnostic capacity, especially if the patient was injured, but this would not have been described as 'advisory' as it also involved treatment, and thus went beyond the limits of what was merely 'advice'. Similarly an apothecary's wares were not necessarily obtained on account of a doctor's 'advice': certain medicines were obtained directly from apothecaries by plague victims' helpers, and readers of self-help books, in addition to the self-diagnostic trend of 'every-housewife-her-own-physician' urged on early modern women by books like *The ladies cabinet* or the Coun-tess of Kent's *Choice manual*, which went through many editions.[45]

These ambiguities of medical 'advice' bring us to the wider question of medical attendance: which practitioners came face to face with their patients as opposed to merely dispensing drugs or giving advice from afar? This is a more complicated question than merely analysing who was giving advice, for it requires a range of indicators to be considered, from specific refer-ences to practitioners visiting the dying at home to more subtle points, such as specifying the fact that the practitioner personally administered physic to the dying individual. Taken together, these indicators appear sufficiently frequently to support a confident assertion that the majority of seventeenth-century practitioners who gave advice to the seriously ill and dying did so in person, certainly after 1660.

Some practitioner designations are obviously very rarely associated with attendance. There are only two instances of men designated 'apothecary' explicitly 'visiting' their patients before 1649, a feature that corresponds well with apothecaries rarely being associated with giving 'advice'. Similarly only two accounts record payments to apprentices or assistants attending or administering physic to the dying person, as opposed to the practitioner

---

[45] Sawyer quotes modern research into medical processes in the Far East which suggest that 93% of all sickness episodes are treated within the family, and 73% of all sickness episodes are only treated within the family: 'Patients, healers', 178.

Table 38
Designations of East Kent practitioners attending the dying in person

	1570–1649	1660–1719
Apothecary	2	6
Doctor	15	222
Physician	36	152
Surgeon	48	48
Not stated	29	301
Total	130	729

himself.[46] By contrast, there is evidence that in more than 50 per cent of cases 'surgeons' were personally attending their patients, and at least 60 per cent of 'physicians' were doing the same after 1660. While this in itself proves nothing other than a greater propensity for accountants and clerks to describe visiting practitioners as 'physicians' and 'surgeons' (regardless of the practitioner's own preferred medical identity), it does correlate with the previous assessment of practitioners' advisory roles. Indeed, the designations assigned to those attending and those giving advice only differ significantly in that a much higher proportion of those attending the dying in the earlier decades were designated 'surgeons', who were comparatively rarely paid for giving 'advice'.

This raises an important point. The medicalisation of serious illness in East Kent over the seventeenth century involved the increased attendance of practitioners at the bedside. The minimum attendance figures of 55 per cent (Status groups A, B and R) and 47 per cent (Status groups C, D and S) in the period after 1660 suggest a very significant increase from the minimum figures of 22 per cent and 14 per cent respectively for before the Civil Wars (see table 42). In addition to these figures, the wider distribution of practitioners after 1660 – and thus the greater physical proximity to rural patients – may be counted as circumstantial evidence that practitioners were more closely associated with their potential patients. It is thus not unreasonable to suggest that practitioners in the later seventeenth century in East Kent far more regularly attended the dying in person than their late sixteenth- and early seventeenth-century counterparts.

---

[46] These are 'paid to the Doctors man for tending him the said deceased' (PRC 2/29/37, dated 1628) and 'to the said Mr Gill's man for his paynes taken about the ministring of the said phisicke' (PRC 2/33/12, dated 1635).

Surgery

The early dictionary compilers (including Blount) do not define 'surgery'. Phillips included it under 'chirurgery' in his *New world of words* (1st edn, 1657) as 'the art of curing wounds', a definition repeated in Elisha Coles's *English dictionary* (2nd edn, 1685). By the eighteenth century the broader concept had found its way into Dr Johnson's dictionary, the definition in his quarto abstract being 'the act of curing by manual operation' (7th edn, 1783). This emphasises the manipulation (instrumental or otherwise) of the body but still does not touch on the treatment by ointments and salves which formed part of the surgeon's art in the seventeenth century.

References to 'surgery' are rarer in the probate accounts than those to 'medicines', 'physic' and 'advice'. Most life-threatening situations, especially with respect to the aged, were not matters which were perceived as being corrected by surgical means. Against this some surgical incisions may have resulted in the deaths of patients here represented, and obviously the emphasis on the treatment of wounds means that a number of those who died of accidents or injuries received surgical attention. The aspects of 'surgery' which appear in the accounts are of four kinds:

1. Cosmetic healing during or after an illness which left visible signs, especially plague and smallpox, usually in respect of surviving members of the family (not the deceased), for example 'to a Chirurgion for healing & curing the aforesayde Agnes Copper daughter of the saide deceased of eyther a plague sore or some other infirmitie which shee had'.[47]
2. The treatment of injuries after a wound, fall or other fatal accident, for example 'paid to the Chyrurgion for searching & dressing the wound of the said deceased he being shott with a peece, whereof he died'.[48]
3. Physical relief which might have equally been provided by an apothecary or physician but which was termed 'surgery' by the accountant as it was provided by a surgeon with a clear occupational identity, for example 'paide to John Russell of Canterburie chirurgion for phisicke or surgerie done to the saide testatorix in the tyme of her sicknes wherof shee dyed'.[49]
4. Other alleviation of ailments probably incidental – or only partly related – to the underlying cause of death, for example 'to John Beeching of the same barber-Chirurgion for his chirurgery and paynes taken to helpe the said deceaseds sore legs'.[50]

As a result the range of surgical functions represented in the accounts is limited, and any conclusions drawn must be regarded as only tentative

---

47 PRC 2/17/292.
48 PRC 20/2/527.
49 PRC 2/13/42.
50 PRC 19/1/47.

Table 39
'Surgery' according to practitioner description in East Kent

	1570–1649	1660–1719
Apothecary	2	0
Barber surgeon	1	0
Physician	1	2
Surgeon	48	6
Not specified	27	4
Totals	79	12

Note: 'Surgeon' includes 'Surgeon and doctor' and 'Surgeon and physician'.

in respect of surgery generally, especially as licensed surgeons were more numerous than other types of officially recognised practitioner.

An important point to make about surgery is that there is a closer relationship between it and its related occupational epithet 'surgeon' than with any other aspect of medicine and associated practitioner designation represented in these accounts. Whereas 'medicines' may be associated with all practitioner designations, and 'advice' may also be regularly connected with all the main designations apart from 'apothecary', 'surgery' is almost exclusively associated with 'surgeon' (see table 39). This does not mean that everyone who performed a surgical act thought of himself or herself as a surgeon – several apothecaries were also licensed surgeons – but to the patient and his family someone performing a surgical act could and should be described as a surgeon.

In fact the correlation of 'surgery' with 'surgeons' is even closer than indicated. Of the thirty-one cases of surgery listed as 'not specified' in table 39, twenty-one practitioners are named and an occupational designation may be applied to most of them on the basis of licensing and similar records. One man, Walter Southwell, was both a freeman apothecary and licensed surgeon; another, Charles Annott, was a freeman surgeon; six others were licensed surgeons; one described himself as a surgeon when signing another surgeon's application for a licence; and three are to be found in other accounts: two as 'surgeons' and one as a 'barber-surgeon'. Discounting the remaining nine (two of whom were women) and regarding the one surgeon-apothecary as an apothecary (so as not to overstate his surgical identity), it is clear that well over 90 per cent of 'surgery' was ascribed to a 'surgeon'.

With regard to the dying, 'surgery' noticeably declines in importance as a term for describing medical intervention after 1660. The word is much more infrequently used. It is possible that the predominance of practitioners being called 'doctor' or 'physician' by the accountants disinclined them to record that such practitioners were paid for 'surgery', or it might be that the term was more narrowly conceptualised at that time, being used only when specifically relating to incision. But it is probable that the terms 'physician' and 'doctor' were becoming more widely regarded as catch-all terms, and many men licensed for surgery were being described as doctors. It is therefore more likely that their services after 1660 were being interpreted in the light of the wider medical remit associated with their popular designation.

Bloodletting

Bloodletting is the only type of treatment usually recognised as surgical which is regularly specified in the probate accounts. It is not possible to determine how much it features as an element of surgery generally, and thus it is not considered in the table and figures above. Evidently it was not the exclusive preserve of the surgeon. Of the forty-one recorded instances of bloodletting, either by itself or in conjunction with another service (for example the administration of medicines), three were associated with a 'doctor' or 'physician', seventeen were associated with a 'surgeon', and twenty-one were not specifically associated with any type of practitioner. Fourteen of the twenty-one unspecified practitioners are named: of these three were licensed surgeons, one was a freeman barber-surgeon licensed to perform surgery and four appear described in other accounts: one as a doctor, one as a physician, one as a physician and apothecary (in separate accounts), and the fourth as a surgeon. Five appear in no other medical context, although one 'Mr Annott' of Canterbury, could be a freeman barber-surgeon (Charles Annott) or a practitioner licensed by the archbishop to perform both medicine and surgery (Peter Annott).

One point which needs to be added is that there is reason to suspect that some of those with no designation were not medical practitioners. Several do not appear in any other context, whether as officially recognised practitioners or in other accounts. Thus although the ratio of physicians to surgeons in letting blood is ostensibly 6:22, it is probable that, as found in other studies, non-practitioners (such as servants) were also undertaking this activity.[51] Indeed, this group is likely to be significantly under-represented in the probate accounts for, if servants and household members were letting blood, they would be unlikely to be paid specifically for the service over and above their wages.

Although the cost of bloodletting with respect to the full range of individuals represented in these accounts is not certain, the prices paid in some instances and with respect to some individuals can be established. This makes it possible to see whether the range of practitioners was mirrored in the range of costs associated with what was otherwise a relatively clearly defined service.[52] It seems that the service, which obviously involved the attendance of

---

[51] Sawyer, 'Patients, healers', 100.
[52] For a full list of bloodletting descriptions found in these accounts see Mortimer, 'Medical assistance', ii. 62.

the person letting the blood and thus often expenses for travel in addition to the actual letting, usually entailed a cost of about 2s. or 2s. 6d. Costs solely for bloodletting (as nearly as can be established) in East Kent include the 2s. 6d. paid in 1636 to William Fox, a Canterbury surgeon, by a Canterbury resident, the 2s. paid in 1618 to Henry Wilford by a fellow parishioner of Milton, and the 2s. paid to a surgeon by a resident of Tenterden – a town with a good complement of practitioners, so very probably a local surgeon – in 1682. Payments above this level tended to include travel, such as the 6s. paid in 1683 by a Frinstead accountant 'to Mr Bayly of Milton for letting the said deceased bloud and for his journey'. The most expensive bloodletting and journey was 10s. paid to Mr Robert Genner in 1681. Payments of 10s. and above were normally associated with other medical fees, such as the 10s. 'to Davison of Staplie Chirurgion for debt due and owinge vnto him by the said deceased at the time of his death for letting him blood & other phisick' in 1618. Most of the payments to named practitioners of less than 3s. are to individuals who are not known to have acted in any other medical capacity. This suggests that local bloodletters were not men with highly developed or widespread practices. Further support for this line of thinking is that the lowest payments for bloodletting – two of 6d. – and several of the payments of less than 4s. do not mention the practitioner by name at all. Thus it seems that not only was there a correlation between fees for the service and practitioner status, as would be expected, but low-status bloodletters only operated within a small locality, and normally catered to the less well-off. From the handful of payments for letting blood in other counties these generalisations seem to reflect the probable situation there too: the amount paid for bloodletting in Berkshire in 1669 being 3s. 6d., and in Sussex in 1635 4s., except where travel expenses brought this figure up, as in the 10s. paid in 1666 to 'Mr Higgs of Wellhouse for lettinge the deceaseds bloud in his lifetime & comeinge up & douwne to him' by a resident of Aldworth, Berkshire.[53]

Medical services in relation to status

In chapter 1 it was shown that there was only a slight difference between the propensity of the higher and lower status groups to adopt a medical strategy to cope with failing health. But this simple comparison ignores the fact that there were probably considerable variations in the types of medical strategy adopted. On the whole it is not possible to determine the quality of care – whether the wealthy received better advice than the poor – but it is possible to investigate the medical services obtained for each group.

There was little difference between the types of services purchased by the higher and lower status groups. This is not in itself surprising: social

[53] BRO, D/A1/188/74A.

Table 40
Status-related descriptions of practitioners paid

| | 1570–1649 | | 1660–1719 | |
| | A, B, R | C, D, S | A, B, R | C, D, S |
	%	%	%	%
Apothecaries	14	11	8	6
Doctors	9	6	29	22
Physicians	16	11	17	17
Surgeons	13	12	7	6
Other specified	1	1	0.1	0.1
Total of unspecified	46	59	40	48
Of those unspecified				
for 'physic'	32	37	32	38
for 'physic and surgery'	1	0.4	0.2	0.1
for medicines	3	3	2	1
for surgery	1	4	1	2
for 'advice' only	0.6	0	0.2	0
for other services	8	15	4	6

Note: Surgery includes bloodletting. Percentages above 1% have been rounded to nearest whole figure.

'superiors' often set the example which the lower status groups followed and, given our reliance on medical occupations, lower status groups may have accorded their practitioners the title of 'doctor' on the basis that that was how the higher status groups chose to describe their practitioners. This would obviously result in parallel descriptions. Some differences, however, may be noted (*see* table 40).

In both the periods 1570–1649 and 1660–1719 the higher status groups were more specific in their application of practitioner descriptions than their lower status contemporaries. While it would be wrong to assume that a lack of precise description implies a lower quality of care, examination of the accounts shows that greater precision was frequently included as a way of justifying higher expense. Examination of the amounts paid 'for physic' by groups A/B/R compared to C/D/S show that in each period and for every type of medical practitioner the amount paid by the wealthier groups was more than that paid by the less well-off groups. Overall, the wealthier groups paid 1.82 times as much as the poorer groups. This is perhaps a surprisingly small difference, considering that groups A/B/R had an average gross estate value more than five times that of status groups C/D/S.

There is no guarantee that seventeenth-century patients received good value for money. Cheap medicine may or may not have been as efficacious as expensive care. As travel was often included in a payment for a practitioner, it might be postulated that the wealthier paid more merely to draw their

Table 41
Payments solely for 'physic' according to practitioner description in East Kent

Status A, B, R	1570–1619 No.	Price (s)	1620–49 No.	Price (s)	1660–89 No.	Price (s)	1690–1719 No.	Price (s)
'Apothecary'	11	19.6	13	43.0	10	31.4	5	30.2
'Doctor'	3	13.0	10	82.8	85	42.4	46	36.4
'Physician'	6	13.9	21	18.8	55	37.5	4	80.3
'Surgeon'	2	12.5	2	25.0	3	50.0	7	37.4
Not specified	32	19.2	72	24.1	150	22.7	88	38.1
Total & avg	54	18.1	118	30.2	303	31.5	150	38.4
Status C, D, S								
'Apothecary'	12	7.9	22	19.5	11	26.7	1	23.8
'Doctor'	7	11.6	13	10.9	70	22.1	23	22.4
'Physician'	8	10.2	26	17.6	33	22.2	0	–
'Surgeon'	–	–	4	12.5	3	16	4	19.9
Not specified	76	10.3	136	14.9	167	16.3	45	19.5
Total & avg	103	10.1	201	15.4	284	18.8	73	20.5
Differences, A, B, R/C, D, S		1.79	–	1.96	–	1.67	–	1.87

Note: The 1620–49 payments to 'doctors' includes one payment of £20 and one of £10.

practitioners from further afield, or more immediately to their bedside, or, as Margaret Pelling has pointed out, more exclusively to their assistance.[54] However there are other qualitative factors which may be considered. Regularity of attendance is one gauge. In the period 1570–1649 the minimum A, B and R attendance rate was more than half as much again as the C, D and S attendance rate (22 per cent compared to 14 per cent) (see table 42). After the Restoration this difference narrowed but was still noticeable (55 per cent to 47 per cent). Furthermore, we can rule out the possibility that the variation in costs on behalf of higher and lower status patients is attributable to the distances travelled by practitioners. Those visiting the lower status groups travelled almost as far – and before 1650 further – than those visiting the higher status groups. Nevertheless the amounts paid by the higher status groups for practitioners' attendance are very much greater than those paid by the lower, whether the practitioner was attending or not.

The assumption that there was a difference in the type of care purchased by those of higher status appears to be supported by this financial differ-

[54] M. Pelling, *Medical conflicts in early modern London: patronage, physicians, and irregular practitioners, 1550–1640*, Oxford 2003, 251–2.

Table 42
Regularity of attendance and costs of medical care in East Kent

Status A, B, R	No.	1570–1649 Avg dist. of patient from town	Cost (s)	No.	1660–1719 Avg dist. of patient from town	Cost (s)
Administering medicines	18	2.2	16.5	270	2.9	37.4
Specified attending	15	1.4	110.2	52	3.1	44.3
Specified visiting	38	2.1	58.4	106	3.1	56.7
Attendance implied	18	3.2	32.2	11	3.4	36.5
Lack of evidence	321	2.1	28.3	369	2.8	37.8
Min. total attend	**22%**				**55%**	

Status C, D, S	No.	Avg dist.	Cost (s)	No.	Avg dist.	Cost (s)
Administering medicines	16	2.4	12.3	180	2.4	21.7
Specified attending	6	1.7	34.4	48	2.4	28.3
Specified visiting	11	2.2	12.5	51	2.1	28.3
Attendance implied	8	3.1	14.3	11	2.6	14.0
Lack of evidence	262	2.4	16.1	328	2.4	20.8
Min. total attend.	**14%**				**47%**	

ence. It could be argued that practitioners charged according to the patient's ability to pay; but even if they did it is likely that the greater ability to pay not only resulted in a higher fee but a higher quality service, according to contemporary perceptions. Ronald Sawyer, in describing a day in the practice of Richard Napier, notes that common people consulting the physician only saw him for a short period whereas a gentlewoman received two hours of his time.[55] Similarly, in respect of a medicine against the plague, Napier drew up two recipes: one for the rich and one for the poor. Thus individual practitioners may consciously have offered differing qualities of service according to a patient's status. Unfortunately the Kent accounts only indirectly reflect this. It is certain that medical care for higher status individuals in East Kent was more expensive, more regularly defined by reference to a commonly recognised occupational epithet, and probably more frequently accompanied by the practitioner's presence than assistance to lower status individuals. But beyond this all that can be done is to investigate whether the same medical practitioners (and thus the same knowledge bases) were serving the wealthy and the poor alike.

[55] Sawyer, 'Patients, healers', 207–11.

The relevance of these findings to the rest of the provincial south of the country is hard to ascertain. There are only twenty-two recorded cases of payments for 'medicine' or 'physic and advice' in Berkshire and West Sussex prior to the Interregnum. Of these, ten are to practitioners of an uncertain designation, and eight of the remaining twelve are specifically to 'apothecaries'. The same proportion is noticeable for the later part of the century: four out of six designated practitioners paid for medicines were 'apothecaries'. The static nature of minimum medical practitioner attendance in these two counties is noteworthy: a constant 7 per cent of males demonstrably receiving attendance in person: 5/72 in the earlier period, and 7/97 in the latter. The other aspect which is touched upon above for East Kent and for which some evidence is available for Berkshire and West Sussex is practitioner nomenclature. Since this subject is treated in greater depth in the next chapter, it is discussed in the overall comparison presented there.

As a result of the thin data for Berkshire and West Sussex, conclusions are based on East Kent data alone. But a number of important points can be made with confidence for this diocese. It would appear that the large increases in the use of medical services by the dying were not accompanied by a commensurate growth in the number of practitioners. In fact it would appear very likely that there was no increase in practitioners at all. This suggests that the nature of medical care to the dying was changing (a supply-side shift) in response to an increase in demand for medical intervention. There can be no certainty about the social changes which wrought these developments in medical practices, but several points are pertinent. First, it has long been known that the seventeenth century was the period in which chemical medicines became widely available, and it is possible that these became the 'new medicine' which allowed practitioners to treat patients more quickly, and which in turn forced them to discard some of the older astrological and less physical aspects of their practices. Second, it is noticeable that practitioners were more frequently living in rural areas: not just outside towns but further from them. Third, medical identities were becoming looser, allowing a greater flexibility of service, so that physicians and surgeons increasingly distributed medicines themselves, taking on a proportion of the urban apothecary's work in the parishes outside towns. Finally, the physicians and surgeons in question, whether rural or urban, were almost certainly attending the dying with greater frequency, thus bringing medicine into the communities, making people aware of medicine, advertising their services and building up their own networks of clients. Any sense that only the wealthy might summon a practitioner in a dire or near-death situation had gone by the end of the seventeenth century: it was a regular occurrence, even for those families who could hardly afford it.

4

Medical Practices

It is no easy task to treat practitioners systematically according to occupation. Not only did some cross between occupations, the historian has also to contend with the fundamental problem of whether to examine the practitioner in the context of the descriptors applied by his clientele, or the identity that he might have assigned to himself, perhaps as a result of a specific qualification. Neither perspective can be ignored. Moreover, the changes in nomenclature and the differences between practitioners' own identities and those assigned to them accentuate the relevance of occupational descriptors. Thus it is worth examining practices according to the practitioners' own and assigned identities, and in the contexts of these to compare their practices in terms of geography and social range, and to see how these may have changed over the period.

The practices of apothecaries

There are 266 specific designations of 'apothecary' in the probate accounts.[1] Of these 158 include the apothecary's name, so that it is possible to look for examples whereby a picture might be built up of the range of geographical and social markets served, and the services rendered by individuals who were referred to as 'apothecaries' on at least an occasional basis. This is supplemented by those who were not referred to as apothecaries in the probate accounts but who were otherwise designated as such (for example in their own probate documents or in records of freemen) and whose practices are also reflected in the probate accounts.

At least twenty-two of the twenty-seven Canterbury apothecaries named in these accounts were freemen of the city.[2] These represent just over half of the forty-two apothecaries granted their freedom in the period 1570–1720. Four of the five who appear in the accounts as apothecaries but who were not freemen are named only once, and the fifth (who may have been a freeman and alderman) is mentioned only twice. In contrast most of the freemen

---

[1]   This includes five entries in accounts dating from the 1720s.
[2]   This does not include George Young, Jr, who may have been the Dr Young who attended a Deal patient nearly forty years after receiving his freedom. A twenty-eighth freeman apothecary, Henry Raworth, was resident in Dover. For a full list see Mortimer, 'Medical assistance', ii. 79–80.

apothecaries are mentioned many times each. This is not surprising: the city authorities could be expected to take action against an apothecary acting illegally on a regular basis. Thus to all intents and purposes any discussion of the Canterbury apothecaries named in the probate accounts is a discussion of the freemen of the city.

Only three of the Canterbury apothecaries – William Sandford, John Greenleaf and John Woolshaffen – are also described as 'doctor' or 'physician'. Although fifteen freemen also held licences, only four of these were apothecaries. These factors suggest there was little ambiguity about apothecaries' identities in the city, among practitioners or customers. However, when the city apothecaries are compared with those described as apothecaries in other towns, a different pattern emerges. There is a striking difference between the types of qualification borne by the apothecaries in smaller towns compared to the city. All but three of the Canterbury apothecaries relied on their freeman status as their only medical qualification. A similar situation seems to have pertained in Maidstone, the second most significant medical town, where none of the nine practitioners mentioned in these accounts as apothecaries held an ecclesiastical licence, and the only other apothecary identified as resident there (Robert Claringbold) was also unlicensed. But of the twenty-six other named men described as apothecaries in the other towns, thirteen had an ecclesiastical licence, and two others professed an alternative medical identity in either their will or marriage licence papers (one a physician and another a surgeon). Another man, although resident in Dover, was a freeman apothecary of Canterbury (having served his apprenticeship there). One apothecary licensed as a physician did not refer to himself as an apothecary in his will but as a physician, suggesting that it was from his licence that he took his occupational identity, even if he was widely known as an apothecary. It seems that in the two major medical towns (Canterbury and Maidstone) where 'apothecaries' could make a profitable income from selling medicines from their shops, this was the limit of their trade. Elsewhere, in the smaller medical towns, the apothecary's business was more often than not supplemented by his service in another medical capacity. In the smallest medical towns, and the villages, practitioners selling medicines were not described as apothecaries at all but as physicians, doctors or surgeons.

As the role of the apothecary was principally that of providing medicines and drugs, the vast majority of the city and town practitioners' individual payments are similar and predictable: the entry 'paid for physic' appears with monotonous regularity. The variations to be noticed are predicated by the alternative medical occupations of apothecaries in the smaller towns: more small-town apothecaries visited their clients (although they were not normally described as apothecaries when acting in this capacity). George Bailey was paid for travelling to Frinstead to let the blood of a gentleman; Elias Martin of Cranbrook (an apothecary and licensed surgeon) appears described as a 'surgeon' and paid for chirurgical applications. By contrast the only identified case of a Canterbury apothecary being paid for performing an act of surgery was Walter Southwell, who was also a licensed surgeon and presumably was acting in this capacity, not as an apothecary. Some small-town apothecaries who were also licensed practitioners of physic or surgery acted in conjunction with other practitioners. For example, although Randolph Partridge of Dover obtained his licence to practice physic in 1626, in accounts dated 1640 and 1641 respectively he was paid for acting in the capacity of an apothecary to three physicians in one instance and as physician and surgeon in another. Another example is the licensed surgeon William Pye, who in 1639 (the year he received his licence for surgery) was described as the apothecary of Mr Samuel Preston ('his apothecary').[3] Had these references appeared in the accounts of very wealthy patients, they might have suggested that apothecaries acted in a pharmaceutical capacity supporting physicians who served the wealthy and acting as physicians in their own right to the less well-off. But they relate to two individuals of Status D and one of Status B. It rather appears that these entries indicate a business relationship: Mr Preston tended to direct his Faversham patients to obtain medicines from Mr Pye (who was also licensed for surgery), and Dr Goulder directed his Dover prescriptions to Randolph Partridge (who also practised as a physician in his own right).[4] Thus a licensed practitioner in a small town might serve as an apothecary to another physician in addition to managing his own practice as a physician or surgeon.[5]

Chapter 3 touched upon the question of whether the same practitioners were at the service of both high and low status patients. As far as apothecaries' services went, it seems that they were. The social ranges of the apothecaries in city and town were reasonably wide: very few seem to have specialised in serving the rich. Those whose patients' average wealth was greatest also served the less well-off. Randolph Partridge of Dover included among his patients a cordwainer, a maltster, a JP ('jurat'), a gentleman, an innholder and a yeoman. Like most apothecaries, his patients were divided across the status groups. Similarly William Finch of Maidstone supplied medicines to two prosperous victuallers, a relatively poor widow (GEV = £26), a rich mercer (GEV = £3,894), a saddler, a ship's carpenter, an esquire and a yeoman. Joseph Colfe, an alderman of Canterbury, was one of the few who predominantly served the well-off. Ten of his twelve patients were

---

[3] For the relationships between physicians and apothecaries see Sawyer, 'Patients, healers', 120–2. Note that there are very few references in the accounts which directly suggest that such relationships existed in Kent.

[4] Napier was solicited for such business contacts in much the same way: ibid. 120–1.

[5] In addition, practitioners supplied medicines to one another, as evidenced by deceased practitioners' accounts mentioning drugs obtained from other practitioners. One example is the payment by the estate of the deceased Richard Heydon of Minster in Sheppey, surgeon, to George Bailey of Milton for 'drugs had of him by the said deceased being a surgeon' which seem to have been for the benefit of the deceased's occupation, not his health: PRC 2/39/187.

Figure 10
Distances of non-Canterbury patients purchasing medicines or physic from Canterbury apothecaries

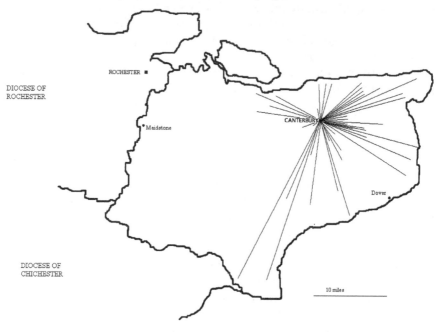

in the top status group. Of the two who were not, one was described as a yeoman and the other, with chattels worth £54, was not in the lowest quartile of wealth represented in these accounts.

Canterbury patients represented a declining proportion of the business of Canterbury practitioners after the Restoration, from 66 per cent to 53 per cent; the apothecaries of other medical towns were serving their own townsmen in 51–2 per cent of cases. But these very similar figures do not reveal the distances being covered by people fetching medicines for those outside the towns. Canterbury was a much stronger magnet for those requiring medical substances than the other towns. A map depicting the range of home parishes of Canterbury apothecaries' customers is strikingly fuller and more far-reaching than that for any of the other smaller towns. In fact it would not be an exaggeration to say that Canterbury dominated the eastern half of the diocese.

With the exception of a handful of long-distance customers, apothecaries based in other medical towns supplied only those within a radius of six miles. Not even Maidstone apothecaries were regularly distributing medicines further afield than this. In his study of early seventeenth-century Buckinghamshire, Ronald Sawyer stressed the importance of major regional centres such as London and Oxford in the supply of medicines; and it could be that

Figure 11
Distances of patients purchasing medicines or physic from Ashford, Dover, Maidstone and Milton/Sittingbourne apothecaries

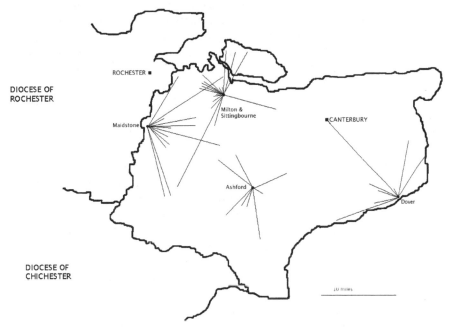

Canterbury should be considered in a similar light. Although there are cases of London apothecaries being paid for medicines, these are only in respect of a few apothecaries' own probate accounts (i.e payments to their wholesale distributors in the capital), and apothecaries' bills satisfied by individuals who died in the capital. East Kent was served by a pharmaceutical centre in Canterbury supported by eight other medical towns with apothecaries' shops. This does not account for the entire supply of medicine in the region, but it establishes the distribution of the services of apothecaries. To obtain medicines other than from these outlets one would have had to get them from a physician, surgeon or grocer, or use the herbs and other easily available medicinal substances which might be found in country gardens.[6]

---

[6]   A grocer was paid for spices in the time of the sickness of Emlyn Heyman of Canterbury (PRC 21/5/98, dated 1581) and one 'Mr Aucher a grocer' was paid 'for necessaries had of him for the said deceased and his children dureing the time he and they lay sicke of the smallpox' in the account of Thomas Ady (PRC 2/41/39, dated 1685). The apothecary Walter Southwell of Canterbury was referred to once in these accounts as a grocer: 'payd to Walter Southwell of the said Citty Grocer for Phisick ministred vnto the sayd deceased': PRC 2/19/163, dated 1620.

The practices of surgeons and physicians

While the definition of 'apothecary' relies predominantly on just two factors – descriptions in account entries (i.e. accountants' perceptions) and the registers of the freemen of Canterbury – the definitions of physicians, doctors and surgeons are more varied and, in consequence, problematic. There are simply too many ways of defining surgeons, doctors and physicians to be able to deal with each exclusively; the varied means of definition result in multiple areas of overlap with regard to qualifications as well as practices, especially after 1660. Although a number of practitioners were unambiguously 'surgeons', the totality of those referred to in some way as 'surgeons' shades rapidly into the ranks of those who practised a range of arts and held a variety of qualifications. So does the totality of 'physicians' and 'doctors'. There were licensed surgeons referred to only as 'physicians' in these accounts, and several practitioners licensed for physic and surgery who cannot easily or correctly be placed exclusively in one camp or the other. While there are a few unambiguous surgeons and a few unambiguous physicians, it is highly unlikely that selection according to consistency of nomenclature would be representative of any group. In addition, it would quite severely limit the sample: of the fifty-six Canterbury practitioners, eighteen were described as 'physician' or 'doctor' without there being any apparent official basis for the practitioner to have such an identity. To eliminate these 'unofficial' individuals from a study of physicians in Canterbury would not only diminish the importance of the accountants' perspective, it would also eliminate one-third of the sample. Thus it seems appropriate to follow both a 'top-down' strategy (based on qualifications and practitioners' self-descriptions), and a separate 'bottom-up' one (based on accountants' perceptions of practitioner identity). Since this dual approach is obviously a complicated exercise, and since the geographical location of each practitioner is not without relevance, the whole sample is divided into geographical sections: Canterbury first, then the major medical towns (which regularly enjoyed the services of an apothecary) then the lesser medical towns (those without designated apothecaries) and finally rural areas.

Canterbury

As with apothecaries, there was a shift among Canterbury practitioners of physic and surgery away from serving their fellow citizens and towards serving the wider community, including rural areas.[7] Moreover, it is noticeable that the increase in the proportion of the Canterbury practitioners' market repre-

---

[7] Four physicians or surgeons were also apothecaries (William Sandford, John Greenleaf, John Woolshaffen and Walter Southwell). However, entries in the accounts relating to these four men show that 30/40 (75%) of the patients naming them were Canterbury

Table 43
Canterbury surgeons for whom evidence of both activity
and occupational identity is available

	Proportion of patients from Canterbury	Avg patient's GEV
1570–1649	37/59 (63%)	£337
1660–1720	24/77 (31%)	£318

Note: Date ranges relate to start of practitioner's career

sented by the population of the diocese outside the city was taking place at a time when the citizens' own use of medical services was increasing rapidly, perhaps doubling. This increase in the use of Canterbury practitioners by non-Canterbury patients is therefore highly significant, remarkable even.

The widest definition which could be applied to the term 'surgeon' would be an all-inclusive one; that is to say any Canterbury practitioner described as a 'surgeon' or 'chirurgion', or any practitioner providing surgery or licensed to practise the art of surgery (whether in conjunction with the art of physic or not) or a freeman surgeon, or a man described in his will as a surgeon. This is the definition used in table 43.

As would be expected, the figures suggest that the people who were paying for the services of named Canterbury surgeons (in the widest definition) were becoming more spread out. After 1660 a significantly higher proportion of patients (almost 70 per cent) did not live within the city. Prior to the Interregnum, people outside Canterbury accounted for just 37 per cent of their cases. The other notable trend is the consistency with which practitioners were described as 'surgeons'. Of the fifteen Canterbury surgeons whose practices were in some way documented before 1650, eight held ecclesiastical licences, three were unlicensed freemen surgeons, and four were 'unqualified'. In the later period all were qualified in some way. Eleven held ecclesiastical licences, three were freemen surgeons or barber-surgeons, and the last was a signatory on an application for a medical licence, so recognised by the authorities as a man of medical reputation in some other way as yet undetermined. But interestingly it was in this later period that the consistency of terminology declined. Apart from late descriptions of Charles Annott as a 'physician' and a single payment to William Fox which describes him as a 'physician', the earlier surgeons were consistently described in the accounts as 'surgeons'. In the later period at least five of the 'surgeons' (William Elvery, Richard Bennister, Peter le Maistre, Peter Morrell and John Woolshaffen) were described as physicians or 'doctors' although they do not

residents, so not counting these four would make the decrease in Canterbury patients as a proportion of the total market even more pronounced.

Table 44
Canterbury physicians for whom evidence of both activity and occupational identity is available

	Proportion of patients from Canterbury	Avg patient's GEV
1570–1649	45/85 (53%)	£369
1660–1720	47/140 (34%)	£364

appear to have possessed qualifications other than those relating to surgery or (in John Woolshaffen's case) pharmacy. It would appear that Canterbury surgeons in general were increasingly being classed alongside physicians in a bracket which denoted medical services in a general sense, and increasingly serving people outside the city.

On the face of it, physicians were, like surgeons, serving more people from outside the city after 1660. However, a close examination of the individuals represented by the above figures shows that after 1660 about half of the physicians were also described as surgeons. In effect half the same group as before is being measured. In theory all those about whom there is the slightest ambiguity could be eliminated, but by so doing half the named physicians in the sample would thereby be eliminated. This is not justifiable: ambiguity of practitioner description was clearly not an aberration but a common feature of the practices of post-1660 practitioners. Moreover the lack of definition in practitioner nomenclature on the part of the clientele, already clear in the case of surgeons, was just as manifest in the descriptions applied to Canterbury physicians. In fact, it was even clearer for, until 1650, whenever the tags of 'physician' and 'doctor' were used in an unofficial way, they related to men who apparently had no qualifications, whereas after 1660 six of the men here described unofficially as a 'physician' or 'doctor' were licensed surgeons. Thus, while a greater proportion of practitioners named in these accounts was in some way officially recognised, the proportion perceived to be doing what they were officially qualified to do was decreasing.

There were some exceptions. To take one of the most eminent physicians represented in these accounts as an example: of the ten accounts which name Sir William Boys (1659–1744), he is described as 'Dr Boys' in nine. The same applies to all those who held a medical doctorate: Ethelbert Spencer (1565–1628) is invariably referred to as 'Dr Spenser'. John Elliot was invariably referred to as Dr Elliot after his award of an MD *per litteras regias* in 1681. William Jacob and William Deeds were also consistently given the pre-title 'Dr'. In those cases where 'Dr' was occasionally not applied, then invariably the epithet 'physician' was added, as with Augustin Caesar and John Peters alias de la Pierre (d. 1688). Consistency of nomenclature for the most highly qualified also applies to those who were licentiates of the

College of Physicians: Jacob Domingo was consistently referred to as 'Dr Thomingo' after his successful altercation with the college in December 1605.[8] The term 'doctor' was consistently applied to all MDs and licentiates of the universities and the college throughout the diocese, not just to the Canterbury practitioners. The same can be said for a number of holders of MB degrees but not all: Thomas Thorpe MB was referred to as Dr Thorpe in only two of the ten payments to him, and Samuel Hall MB in only one of his seven payments.

Other major medical towns

In East Kent the designation 'apothecary' can be related exclusively to only nine of the 'medical towns' initially identified in chapter 1. In addition, closer scrutiny of the most significant of these towns reveals that there were important differences between the largest nine or ten – where inhabitants showed a high degree of loyalty to their local practitioners – and the rest, where inhabitants tended to seek medical help elsewhere more often than they sought it from their home town. For these two reasons the 'major medical towns' here are those which were the most medically populated and which had practitioners who were regularly described as 'apothecaries', namely Maidstone, Dover, Sittingbourne and Milton-next-Sittingbourne (treated as one), Faversham, Ashford, Sandwich, Cranbrook and Tenterden.

Tables 45 and 46 show that the pattern of towns catering to a wider hinterland – so clearly observable in Canterbury – was not followed in every other medical town. Overall the proportion of the market represented by the towns' own inhabitants shrank by about 12 per cent – from about 54 per cent to about 42 per cent – less than Canterbury (where it declined from about 57 per cent to 35 per cent). But Dover in particular displayed a markedly different pattern. There the local clientele as a proportion of the practitioners' market began very high (74 per cent) and increased to 82 per cent. Similarly Maidstone did not see a 10 per cent decrease; rather it remained stable at about 42 per cent. Faversham and Sittingbourne residents also continued to represent a significant portion of their local practitioners' market.

Exactly why there was a diversity of experience in the towns is not clear. Individual factors seem to have affected each town differently. A diminution in the town's population, such as happened in Sandwich over the early part of the seventeenth century, for example, may well have forced practi-

8 According to *The roll of the Royal College of Physicians of London compiled from the annals of the college and from other authentic sources*, ed. W. Munk, London 1861, in December 1605 Domingo was accused of practising without licence by the college, and, after revealing evidence showing him to be an extra-licentiate of the college, was given a full licence. See also Pelling, *Medical conflicts*, 243.

Table 45

Practices of physicians and surgeons in the major eight medical towns
outside Canterbury, 1570–1650

Town	Patients from same town	Status A, B, R patients from same town	Status C, D, S patients from same town	Mean GEV
Ashford	12/32 (37.5%)	3/11	9/21	£210
Cranbrook	2/3 (67%)	1/2	1/1	£370
Dover	23/31 (74%)	9/11	14/20	£126
Faversham	9/19 (47%)	1/6	8/13	£165
Maidstone	12/28 (43%)	2/10	10/18	£153
Sandwich	30/47 (64%)	14/23	16/24	£202
Sittingbourne and Milton	7/22 (32%)	3/12	4/10	£231
Tenterden	14/21 (67%)	10/14	4/7	£527
Totals	109/203 (54%)	43/89	66/114	£221

Table 46

Practices of physicians and surgeons in the major eight medical towns
outside Canterbury, 1660–1720

Town	Patients from same town	Status A, B, R patients from same town	Status C, D, S patients from same town	Mean GEV
Ashford	14/67 (21%)	8/39	6/28	£251
Cranbrook	6/17 (35%)	3/13	¾	£367
Dover	28/34 (82%)	14/18	14/16	£221
Faversham	48/90 (54%)	30/58	18/32	£240
Maidstone	21/50 (42%)	13/34	8/16	£353
Sandwich	26/72 (36%)	12/44	14/28	£257
Sittingbourne and Milton	27/74 (36%)	13/41	13/32	£232
Tenterden	3/11 (27%)	3/8	0/3	£139
Totals	173/415 (42%)	96/255	76/159	£266

tioners based there to establish new markets further afield.[9] A significant
increase in the town's size, on the other hand, as at Maidstone, might have
provided established practitioners with sufficient business not to need to
travel out of the town. This might explain why the Maidstone figures are

9 For the reduction in the population of Sandwich see Bower, 'Kent towns', 160.

static throughout.[10] In addition increasing numbers of rural practitioners may have cornered the business in some rural areas, to the detriment of some towns, but not others. For example, practitioners resident in Sandwich may have looked upon Thanet as part of their hinterland before medical practitioners regularly took up residence there. Differences in regional wealth may also have affected medical markets: it might not be a coincidence that practitioners in Dover, who served more of their fellow townsmen than any other town, also catered for the poorest people (by average) in the pre-1650 period and the second poorest after the Restoration.

Having made these points it should be reiterated that overall the external shifting of the market noticed in Canterbury is broadly reflected in the totality of major medical towns and with regard to lower as well as higher status groups. The same can also be said of the other features noted for Canterbury: the proportion of named practitioners who were qualified in some way increased, albeit slightly; and a greater inconsistency of description was reflected in the terms applied to practitioners, especially surgeons, after 1660. It would appear that before the end of the century the term 'doctor' was practically synonymous with 'physician' and both words could be applied to any medical practitioner recognised officially as having a variety of medical skills (therefore including surgeons but excluding bloodletters). Charles Goodall in London was perhaps right when he accused many county practitioners of calling themselves 'doctor' without official approbation; he would certainly have been right if he had stated that their patients called them 'doctors'. But he was wrong to think that this was solely the fault of the practitioners themselves or that there could be any return to the old definition of the word, whereby only holders of doctorates were 'doctors'. The popular growth of medical assistance over the seventeenth century had resulted in a popularisation of the terminology. Nor was Goodall right to assume all these new 'doctors' were merely self-taught quacks; several had licences to practise surgery, obtained after examination by their peers, and so had at least an acceptable base of contemporary orthodox medical knowledge.

Lesser medical towns

The places which have not so far been mentioned were a mixture of small urban settlements and rural parishes. Several of the medical towns in East Kent (Deal, Elham, Hythe, Lydd and New Romney, Wye and, for a restricted area, Lenham) do not seem to have offered the services of an apothecary during this period. Thus they may be referred to as lesser medical towns, a designation supported by their minor importance in providing medical services to their own inhabitants and their hinterlands (see table 14).

---

[10] For the increase in the population of Maidstone see ibid. According to Bower Maidstone doubled in population between 1560 and 1640.

Table 47
Qualifications and consistency of description of surgeons from Canterbury and the principal eight other medical towns

Town	Period into which practitioner's career predominantly falls	Practitioners licensed or officially recognised	Practs licensed only for surgery but described as 'physician' or 'doctor'
Ashford	1570–1650	8/10	0/2
"	1660–1720	5/7	1/2
Cranbrook	1570–1650	2/2	0/1
"	1660–1720	3/3	0/1
Dover	1570–1650	6/7	0/3
"	1660–1720	5/7	3/4
Faversham	1570–1650	3/8	0/2
"	1660–1720	8/8	0/2
Maidstone	1570–1650	7/10	5/6
"	1660–1720	8/12	2/4
Sandwich	1570–1650	6/13	0/5
"	1660–1720	5/8	1/1
Sittingbourne and Milton	1570–1650	4/5	–
"	1660–1720	11/13	3/6
Tenterden	1570–1650	3/4	0/1
"	1660–1720	1/3	–
Totals	1570–1650	39/59 (66%)	5/20 (25%)
"	1660–1720	46/60 (77%)	11/20 (55%)
Canterbury	1570–1650	19/31 (61%)	2/7 (29%)
"	1660–1720	25/26 (96%)	6/12 (50%)

It is at this level that the limitations of the geographical aspects of the sources, especially licensing records, are exposed. Of the sixty-nine practitioners who may be associated with the lesser medical towns, thirty-five are represented in the accounts. However, none of the ten practitioners who may be associated with Wye is mentioned. Nor is there any evidence that Wye residents obtained their medical services locally; their practitioners were normally sought in or from Ashford. This can only be explained by suggesting that licensing records often related to the applicants' parishes of origin, not necessarily the place where they practised. In support of this it is noticeable that several East Kent practitioners received their licences as of one place, and then appear in the accounts as of another.

This suggests that some of the so-called lesser medical towns might simply have been places where, in the early seventeenth century especially, men emerged with an education and ambition to become practitioners elsewhere, in the most important medical towns. Only Hythe was the medical focus for more than ten patients whose accounts name a practitioner before the Interregnum. However, these towns do seem to have grown significantly in importance, and while they may be separated from the major medical towns by the absence of designated apothecaries, their importance in the supply of medical services undeniably grew over the century. Apart from Deal, the degree to which the lesser medical towns served their hinterlands was comparable with the major medical towns; and the regularity with which men officially licensed for surgery were described as physicians and doctors is comparable. The proportion of practitioners qualified in some way or other also is comparable. The differences between the lesser medical towns and the major ones in 1700 were that the hinterlands of the lesser medical towns were smaller in size, the patients using them were generally less wealthy, there was only one medical degree-holder to be found in any of them (Isaac Warquin) and the most common qualification found there – the diocesan licence to practise surgery – was even more frequently the sole qualification borne by a 'physician' or 'doctor'.

Table 48
Practices of physicians and surgeons in the lesser medical towns, 1570–1650

Town	Patients from same town	Status A, B, R patients from same town	Status C, D, S patients from same town	Mean GEV
Deal	1/5	1/2	0/3	£121
Elham	1/2	–	1/2	£46
Hythe	4/16	3/5	1/11	£84
Lydd and New Romney	5/6	2/3	3/3	£146
Lenham	1/3	1/2	0/1	£144
Totals	12/32 (37.5%)	7/12	5/20	£103

Note: One case has been excluded from the GEV for Lydd and New Romney, as it was £4,851, which skews the rest of the sample. If it were to be included the GEV average would be £930.

Table 49
Practices of physicians and surgeons in the lesser medical towns, 1660–1720

Town	Patients from same town	Status A, B, R patients from same town	Status C, D, S patients from same town	Mean GEV
Deal	19/22 (86%)	11/14	8/8	£168
Elham	10/42 (24%)	6/21	4/21	£196
Hythe	8/36 (22%)	5/21	3/15	£163
Lydd and New Romney	11/23 (48%)	6/11	5/12	£167
Lenham	1/2	1/1	0/1	£135
Totals	49/125 (40%)	29/68	20/57	£175

Table 50
Qualification and consistency of description of surgeons for lesser medical towns

Town	Period into which practitioner's career predominantly falls	Practitioners licensed or officially recognised	Practs licensed only for surgery but described as 'physician' or 'doctor'
Deal	1570–1650	1/1	0/1
"	1660–1720	5/8	3/3
Elham	1570–1650	1/1	0/1
"	1660–1720	3/4	2/3
Hythe	1570–1650	4/4	3/4
"	1660–1720	4/5	3/4
Lydd and New Romney	1570–1650	2/4	0/2
"	1660–1720	3/4	1/2
Lenham	1570–1650	0/2	–
"	1660–1720	0/1	–
Totals	1570–1650	8/12	3/8
"	1660–1720	15/22	9/12

Rural parishes

There are seventy-three other parishes in East Kent with which a practitioner can be associated. The predominant sources for drawing up this list
are the diocesan and archiepiscopal registers of licences, and thus a possible
reason for there being no payments in the accounts associated with physicians and surgeons in thirty-four of these parishes is that, as suggested above,
the parish noted relates to the paternal home of a young man who moved
away when licensed to set up his own practice elsewhere.[11] Another reason is
that a number of early seventeenth-century rural licentiates were clergymen
who do not appear in these accounts, perhaps because they treated patients
only rarely but more probably because they did not feel it consistent with
their vocation to make a charge for their services when their patients died.
This leaves thirty-nine rural parishes that had resident practising physicians
and surgeons. Four of these may be construed as possible 'towns': Appledore
appears described as having a market by Lambarde in 1570, by Norden in
1625 and by the anonymous compiler of the 1662 list; and Lambarde also
notes Smarden and Sutton Valence as having markets in 1570. But Appledore's population was 120 adults in 1676, and the markets in Smarden and
Sutton Valence (the adult populations of which in 1676 were 210 and 224
respectively) do not appear to have lasted into the seventeenth century.[12]
Thus for the purposes of assessing medical geography, these places had more
in common with the parishes that surrounded them than with the medical
towns, even the lesser ones.

Perhaps not surprisingly, the majority of these practitioner-inhabited rural
parishes for which there is evidence of payments are the parishes around
Ashford, the Isle of Sheppey and in the Isle of Thanet.[13] However, not even
the most established rural practitioners appear in these accounts with any
great frequency. By the end of the period in question, practitioners in Thanet
were regularly mentioned in the capacity of serving their own clientele; but
otherwise many references to rural practitioners are one-off payments. This
suggests that most rural medical practices were less far-reaching and less
pervasive than their urban counterparts. But what is particularly interesting
are the social and geographical patterns displayed by those for which there

[11] An unambiguous example is that of Edmund Randolph MD (1602–49), son of Bernard
Randolph of Biddenden, who became a Canterbury physician. Another is that of Ethelbert Spencer MD (1565–1628), son of John Spencer of Chart Sutton, who also moved to
Canterbury. An example of a less prestigious practitioner was Simon Hammond (d. 1703),
who received his licence for surgery in 1675 as 'of Chart Sutton' but who seems to have
practised at Bearsted and was described as 'of Bearsted' in his probate grant.

[12] *Compton Census*, 27, 30. These are specifically male and female populations able to
receive holy communion, and do not include children.

[13] Several practitioners for the Isle of Sheppey have not been included as they cannot
be pinned down to a particular parish, nor can their medical identities be checked in any
way. See surnames Everard, Hunt, Jackson, James and Londey in Mortimer, *Directory*.

Table 51

Social and geographic ranges of East Kent physicians and surgeons, 1570–1649

Hometown of practitioner	Patients from same town	Status A, B, R	Status C, D, S	Mean GEV
Canterbury	66/115 (57%)	52%	62%	£346
Major medical towns	109/203 (54%)	48%	58%	£221
Lesser medical towns	12/32 (37.5%)	58%	25%	£103
Rural parishes	6/36 (17%)	15%	22%	£245

Table 52

Social and geographic ranges of East Kent physicians and surgeons, 1660–1720

Hometown of practitioner	Patients from same town	Status A, B, R	Status C, D, S	Mean GEV
Canterbury	52/149 (35%)	29%	45%	£367
Major medical towns	173/415 (42%)	38%	48%	£266
Lesser medical towns	49/125 (40%)	43%	35%	£175
Rural parishes	32/92 (35%)	29%	44%	£223

are records of activity. Putting this information together with the previous comparable data for the other areas in East Kent where practitioners were situated reveals an obvious trend for rural people to source medical expertise closer to home as well as increasingly from the city and towns.

Physicians and surgeons from Canterbury were increasingly finding their markets outside the city, and those from the major medical towns were doing likewise (with the exception of Dover). But in the country there was a significant upturn in local business as well. Over the period under study, the market seems to have shifted into rural areas, and the major towns seem to have lost what had been (c. 1570–1600) a near monopoly of the supply of occupationally defined medical expertise. It is interesting that the average (mean) wealth of those in rural parishes naming their practitioners dropped, despite the fact that overall the wealth of patients represented in the sample of probate accounts increased very significantly. This must be seen as evidence towards a 'lowering of the drawbridge' in the ability of rural parishioners to obtain medical relief. Overall, practitioners serving the dying in rural areas had almost the same client base as Canterbury practitioners in the period 1660–1720, with regard to status and local community. Canterbury practitioners may have been more highly qualified and might have travelled further to see their patients, and their high-status patients

Table 53
Levels of qualification and consistency of surgeons' descriptions in East Kent

	Period into which practitioner's career predominantly falls	Practitioners licensed or officially recognised %	Surgeons described as 'physician' or 'doctor' %
Canterbury	1570–1650	61	29
"	1660–1720	96	50
Major medical towns	1570–1650	66	25
"	1660–1720	76	55
Lesser medical towns	1570–1650	67	37.5
"	1660–1720	68	75
Rural parishes	1570–1650	<65	29
"	1660–1720	<82	60

may have been wealthier, but otherwise the proportion of low-status local cases that they saw was the same as the average practitioner in the country.

Perhaps less surprising are the aspects of nomenclature recorded for rural practitioners. Here the methodology employed so far becomes slightly problematic as the practice of ignoring physicians and surgeons whose home towns cannot be identified means that many practitioners who might have been resident in small towns or rural parishes have had to be ignored. These are frequently practitioners without any known qualification. Consequently the proportion of 'qualified' practitioners recorded in table 53 for rural areas is a maximum, and the true percentage will be lower, possibly much lower. Nevertheless the increase in the proportion of practising rural physicians and surgeons with some form of qualification is noticeably in line with the increase in Canterbury and the major medical towns.

Finally it should be noted that the increasing tendency in all the medical towns to describe practitioners licensed to practice surgery as 'physicians' or 'doctors' is mirrored in the rural parishes. John Smith of St Johns Thanet, an elderly licensed surgeon, was even described explicitly as 'the doctor' in 1668, suggesting a uniquely identified community-bound role akin to that of 'the rector' or 'the lord of the manor'.[14] Across the whole diocese, of all 106 practitioners licensed only for surgery, the proportions described in the accounts as doctors or physicians increased from 11/42 (26 per cent) before

[14] William Philpott of St Johns Thanet 'paid to John Smith the doctor for physick when the said deceased lay upon his death bed': PRC 1/13/91, dated 1668.

the Interregnum to 37/64 (58 per cent) after the Restoration. It may be possible to say that by about 1700 the diocesan licence to practise surgery had effectively become the qualification for 'general practice' in the eyes of the communities served, if not of the practitioners themselves, and this may be said for the city and the medical towns almost as much as for rural areas.

Geographical proximity and practitioner choice

Certain generalisations about the practices and descriptions of physicians and surgeons in East Kent in the seventeenth century may now be made. However, by aiming to establish reliable statements about qualifications and markets for medical services, a number of more subtle distinctions have been glossed over. These concern proximity and exclusiveness, information about which may be extracted from the East Kent model with regard to smaller constituencies of practitioner groups and individual practitioners. Likewise there has been no examination about how these findings affect existing debates about the factors which influenced patients' choice of practitioner, especially the relevance of proximity and the exclusivity of the most highly qualified physicians' practices. These issues now need to be addressed.

To begin with proximity, the traditional view of early modern medical relationships is that the higher the status of the patient, the stronger the relationship with his or her practitioner, and the further that practitioner might be required to travel in order to help the patient. The nobility and higher gentry might summon their practitioners from a distance of a hundred miles, or even more; the lesser gentry might seek help from up to twenty miles away; but most people travelled not much further than the next market town. However, there is little evidence to support these generalisations except private accounts which demonstrate that the wealthiest people did summon their physicians over long distances. The traditional view has largely been accepted on the assumption that the less well-off could not have afforded to do the same, and thus must have followed more modest geo-economic patterns.

The principal exception to this lack of systematic evidence is Ronald Sawyer's work on Napier's practice. Sawyer heavily stresses the importance of proximity. He states that 'the most important factor influencing resort [to a medical practitioner] was simply proximity'.[15] He places this at the top of a general 'hierarchy of resort', followed by (2) 'personal relationship to the healer or neighbours' pattern of consultation'; (3) 'price'; (4) 'type of disease and speciality of healer'; and (5) 'consistency of doctor's ideas and therapeutics with patient's expectations'. These other elements of the hierarchy were, he argues, of differing importance to different individuals, and

---

15 Sawyer, 'Patients, healers', 196.

the sick moved between types of practitioner in a 'frantic shuttle' of medical consumption which 'only cure or death could stop'.[16] However, while he acknowledges that the non-geographical elements in the hierarchy were interchangeable, proximity remains foremost in his analysis, underpinning much of his view of the medical landscape. For him it was the reason why clergymen and gentlewomen played 'a huge role' in the provision of medical care, the great majority of Napier's patients living within ten miles of his house.[17]

Sawyer's analysis of patient choice marks a significant advance in understanding why patients employed particular practitioners. However, there are several problems. The first of these lies in the way he uses Napier's records to determine patient choice. Sawyer presumes that the records of a practitioner reflect the wide variety of influences considered by potential patients. They do not. They are only evidence in so far as they represent the option eventually chosen by patients; they do not reflect the wider decision-making processes. Nor do they offer any details about those who decided not to employ Napier. To use a modern analogy, this is like claiming that all those who invested in one particular company's shares are representative of all financial investors. This can hardly be the case; those who did not employ Napier may have exercised choice in a completely different way.

By stating that proximity was the most important factor in the hierarchy, Sawyer implies that distance was of relevance to most sufferers. Obviously 'important' cannot mean universal pre-eminence in this context, otherwise everyone would have gone to their nearest practitioner. Rather it must be taken to mean that, while proximity may not have been at the top of each individual's personal 'hierarchy of resort', it would have appeared on most people's list of priorities. This raises the question of defining 'proximity'. Sawyer uses 'a ten-mile radius'. No point in East Kent was as much as ten miles from a major medical town; and no major medical town at the start of the seventeenth century had fewer than three practising physicians, with the possible exceptions of Cranbrook and Sittingbourne. Even so, a patient on the far side of Cranbrook would have been within ten miles of Tenterden. A ten-mile radius around a fixed point amounts to an area of 314 square miles (201,061 acres); in East Kent this is about a fifth of the whole county, or one-third of the diocese of Canterbury, and thus within reach of between twenty and seventy medical practitioners. On this basis it cannot be argued that, just because most of Napier's patients came from within ten miles of Great Linstead, proximity was the prime factor influencing patients to go to him. Indeed, if the East Kent findings are used, it can be said that if patients were travelling more than three miles, proximity was clearly not the most

16 Ibid. 201.
17 Ibid. 196.

important factor, as the average non-urban patient in East Kent was about three miles from a medical town.

In the East Kent accounts there is certain evidence of the decisions made by the dying and their relatives, and only limited evidence of the choices they faced prior to making those decisions. This means that, as when assessing Sawyer's conclusion, those aspects of patient choice which appear to be the most widely relevant to us were not necessarily the most important to the patients and their families. For instance, a tendency to obtain medical help from a distance of less than three miles does not in itself mean that proximity was a motivating factor: rather it could be that the practitioners whose reputations were best known to dying patients tended to be local, and the apparent 'importance' of proximity is merely a symptom of the importance of knowing a practitioner's reputation. However, setting such objections aside, all Sawyer's influencing factors are evidenced to a greater or lesser extent in East Kent. Estimations of the relevance of Sawyer's prime factor, proximity, have been made in the sections in chapter 1 dealing with geography. Sawyer's second factor, 'personal relationship to the healer', is more difficult to measure, but is suggested in those East Kent accounts which stress the possessive nature of patients' relationships with their practitioners. For example, the account of Susan Omer of Bekesbourne (1631) records a payment 'to her Phisicion', Dr Leonard of Canterbury, and the account of Daniel Lawrence of Faversham, mariner (1661), mentions a payment 'to Mr David Joanes the deceased's physician for physick administered unto the said deceased ... and for his advice'.[18] At Status D and Status B respectively, these were almost certainly not economically powerful people. Thus, reflecting back on proximity, if relationships of trust could develop in the course of long illnesses among people of no great wealth or influence, it is not justifiable to presume that they would not send for their practitioner even if he were some miles distant. With regard to the second element in this factor – 'neighbours' pattern of consultation' – this may be reflected in local communities seeking assistance from the same practitioners.

Sawyer's third factor, price, is reflected in the fact that higher status individuals paid more for their medicine than those of lower status. However, the difference between the prices paid by higher and lower status groups was not very great and so this may perhaps be considered less important in the context of serious illness and dying patients than otherwise. When facing death, individuals often spent more on medical help than they would normally have done on other services or commodities. Conversely, practitioners sometimes waived fees when their patient died. Nevertheless price cannot be discounted entirely, for the obvious reason that not all practitioners would have regarded all sick people as equally able to pay their fees, and not all sick families would have regarded all practitioners as affordable.

[18] PRC 2/31/53; PRC 1/8/107.

The last two influencing factors, 'type of disease and speciality of healer' and 'consistency of doctor's ideas and therapeutics with patient's expectations', are not unrelated. Although there is little certain evidence regarding the latter, it might be said that employment of a specialist to a great extent conforms to the model of a patient wishing to see his therapeutic expectations fulfilled. Patients in one substantial medical town regularly sought the assistance of a practitioner from another, more distant place. This might have been due to relationships of trust or a prior obligation; however, in most cases it is likely to have been due to medical reputation or perceptions of skill in respect of specific challenges, especially surgical ones. When the prosperous Ashford inn-keeper, James Mascall, had an accident in the 1620s, he not only purchased local expertise (from the wonderfully-named surgeon, Comfort Starr), but sought the assistance of 'Mr Charles Annott of Canterbury Chirurgion for Chirurgicall applicacions by him ministred and applied to the said deceased testator before his death in the tyme he lay greeved and sick with the fall hurt or infirmity wherof he died.'[19] Similarly, when Robert Curtis, gent, of Tenterden was taken ill (and later died) at an inn in New Romney, he sent a messenger to Canterbury and Tenterden to bring four practitioners to him, including Dr Randolph, Charles Annott and Peter Peters of Canterbury, and (Alexander?) Devison from Tenterden. [20] Incidents such as this may well explain why some surgeons and physicians – Mr Charles Annott among them – appear very much more frequently in these accounts than others.

Sawyer's 'hierarchy of resort' may thus be seen to have relevance for the dying but only as a non-hierarchical interdependent series of factors. Proximity was important but not as important as he suggests. Likewise price was less important in serious cases. His work has great value in drawing attention to criteria which were, at some time or other, important in decision-making. But it also requires considerable extension and clarification. For example, 'type of disease and speciality of healer' suggests that patients chose a practitioner according to their ailment; this does not sufficiently stress the ways in which the infectious nature of a disease might restrict the choice of practitioner. Nor does it sufficiently stress the importance of fear – the fear of death, or immobility, or scarring, which accompanied certain diseases – which may well have resulted in a choice of practitioner which was not so much rational (as Sawyer seems to suggest) as desperate. Some individuals had personal reasons for their practitioner choice, for example tenants of property owned by medical practitioners may have felt bound to use the services of their landlord as opposed to other town tradesmen, even against their better judgement. Naval personnel may have felt bound to use service

[19] PRC 2/25/162.
[20] PRC 19/1/36; I. Mortimer, 'The triumph of the doctors: medical assistance to the dying, *c.* 1570–1720', *Transactions of the Royal Historical Society* 6th ser. xv (2005), 97–116 at p. 97.

practitioners, even when not at sea. Physical boundaries (for example the Swale) may have distorted 'proximity' by discouraging patients' representatives from making even short journeys to call upon practitioners, especially in bad or winter weather. Diseases of children may well have inclined patients to seek advice from local women as opposed to a medical practitioner, not only for the women's experience but for fear of embarrassment and unnecessary expense if the ailment turned out to be short-lived or minor. Females may have preferred to consult other women specifically on account of their gender. Religious aspects – the moral respectability of the practitioner and the likelihood of his being a suitable channel for God's healing power – may also have affected choice. Finally, Sawyer's hierarchy assumes universal social inclusiveness on the part of the practitioner. Napier was not dismissive of lower status patients, and consequently Sawyer does not consider social and religious exclusivity in seventeenth-century medicine, as if all practitioners were waiting to receive any sick person who happened to drop by. This may have been the case in early seventeenth-century rural Buckinghamshire, and it may even have been the case in parts of early seventeenth-century Kent, but it would be unrealistic to suggest that class played no part in relationships between patients and practitioners.[21]

Case studies

Case studies are useful in exploring factors, such as the importance of exclusion and proximity, influencing practitioner choice in East Kent. Whereas Sawyer's work does this in respect of a single rural practice, to get a fuller picture it is necessary to compare a variety of urban and rural practices.

Medical degree-holders: exclusivity and range

Those with MD or MB degrees were the most highly qualified practitioners in the diocese. They may also have been the most exclusive. The average GEV of those employing one of the four Canterbury medical degree-holders before 1650 was £425, somewhat in excess of the mean of £347 for anyone employing any designated physician or surgeon from the city, or the £321 GEV of the average 'gentleman' as described in probate accounts dated before 1650. After 1660 the fifty patients employing William Jacob, John Peters, Samuel Hall, Sir William Boys or William Deeds had an average GEV of £461, still considerably higher than the £337 of the average 'gentleman' at that time.

---

[21] Ann Hess's findings with regard to Quaker midwifery support this. Although non-Quaker midwives were employed, they were a minority: 'Midwifery practice among the Quakers in southern rural England in the late 17th century', in Marland, *Art of midwifery*, 53.

Close examination of the individuals' remits suggests caution in assuming exclusiveness, however. While one of Dr Ethelbert Spencer's patients had chattels worth £732, the other three were all Status C patients in the first two decades of the seventeenth century (before the significant increases in medical help to that group are noticeable). Similarly Dr Thomas Leonard's patients included a Status D spinster (GEV £32), and a relatively poor clerk (GEV £42), neither of whom were of Canterbury, as well as prosperous citizens. It may well be that the spinster (Susan Omer) had wealthier connections which helped her in her search for a cure for her 'cancer' (her accountant paid Dr Leonard £11), but nevertheless the tendency for medical degree-holders to assist the less well-off at this time is attested to by other cases too. The Canterbury MD at this time whose patients were by far the wealthiest, with an average estate of £672 (Edmund Randolph), also assisted Status D patients. Amongst the esquires and gentlemen he treated was one John Beale of Biddenden, with chattels worth £29, but he also cared for a Canterbury spinster worth £20, and a grocer of Sandwich worth just £2 (possibly retired and living in someone else's house).

After 1660 it seems that exclusiveness prevailed among this group. Six of Sir William Boys's patients had chattels worth more than £600; the others all had considerably in excess of £200. William Deeds and Samuel Hall are likewise recorded only in the context of Status A patients. The best-represented MD, William Jacob, seems to have been less exclusive, treating a number of Status B patients; but still the majority were Status A, and those of lesser status mostly had some aspect which suggests that their wealth does not fully reflect their connections, such as those specifically of 'no occupation', or the pre-title 'squire'. Dr Peters alone of these MDs assisted patients who could have been of a lowly status, such as Elizabeth Mills, widow of Herne (GEV £36) and Bartholomew Roger of Canterbury (GEV £29) along with his wealthier clientele.

The problem with an impressionistic method of assessing exclusiveness is that we forget how the proportions of higher and lower status individuals are represented in these accounts. For example, the four pre-1649 Canterbury MDs saw seven higher status patients and ten lower status between them. To say then that they saw patients in a ratio of 7:10 does not reflect the fact that for the period 1570–1649 there are 7,297 lower status patients represented in these accounts compared to just 2,170 higher status individuals. Thus it is worth running an adjusted check to see how the impression of increasing exclusivity may be reflected in the proportions of lower status patients gaining access to MDs. This may be done by adjusting the number of lower status patients in proportion to the numbers of accounts extant for each status group, in this case 7297/2170 or 3.36. This makes it possible to quantify a lower status patient's accessibility to medical degree-holders relative to that of a notional higher status patient. Thus for these four Canterbury medical degree-holders in the period 1570–1649 the calculation is $(10/3.36)/7 = 0.42$. This figure serves as an approximate measure of relative accessibility and thus may be compared to the access of lower status patients to medical degree-holders in other periods and places. The relative accessibility of medical degree-holders from outside Canterbury in the same period (including Dr Golder) is $(10/3.36)/10 = 0.30$. In other words, before the Interregnum it was harder for lower status patients to gain access to MDs established outside Canterbury than within the city. After 1660 the ratio of lower status to higher status accounts is 2122/1834 or 1.16. This gives relative accessibility figures of 0.16 for Canterbury medical degree-holders, and 0.30 for medical degree-holders from outside the city. It appears that the impression that the social exclusiveness of Canterbury medical degree-holders greatly increased over the seventeenth century is a justified one, as significantly fewer lower status patients were seen. Medical degree-holders outside the city, however, remained just as accessible to lower status patients as before.

In considering the range of patients seen by these doctors of medicine the obvious next line of enquiry is that of how the cost of their services varied from patient to patient. Unfortunately there is no possibility of using this data in any meaningful way. There are simply too many variables, such as what arrangements already existed between the patients and their doctors, what was wrong with the patients or, even more important, what was thought to be wrong with them. Nor is it possible to establish, in most cases, how much of a fee was charged for travel. To take the patients of John Peters (d. 1688) for example: Thomas Goulding of Seasalter (GEV £32) paid 3s. to Dr Peters for 'physick' and Matthew Chandler of Canterbury (GEV £111) paid 5s. for 'his pains and advice'. Anne Coppin of Thanet, a comparatively wealthy woman with a GEV of £516, also paid just 4s. The comparatively poor Mary Wolrich of Boughton under Blean (GEV £23), on the other hand, paid 15s. for physic and Dr Peters 'coming to visit'. While much of this may have been travel expenses, it was exceeded as an amount by the 20s. paid by Bartholomew Roger of Canterbury (GEV £29), in respect of whom Dr Peters's travel expenses would have been minimal. Another Canterbury man, the cutler William Dollman (with an estate of £421), was much wealthier than Bartholomew Roger, but paid half the fee, 10s. Thus, without further information on what the practitioners actually did, and how they calculated their fees, the amounts paid to them cannot be used to explore how payments might have reflected a patient's ability to pay.

Geographically, the Canterbury MDs covered all of the eastern part of the diocese and strayed into the western half. Just five doctors of medicine could cover a lot of ground (see figure 12). Considering that it shows only thirty-four entries between these five men (sixteen of their patients being Canterbury residents), it is clear that the medical hinterland of the county town was far broader than the six miles used as a measurement in chapter 1. The obvious implication of this is, in terms of medical availability, that the population from which selected patients could be drawn was indeed very much greater than the population of the city in which the practitioners lived. So,

Figure 12
Area covered by three Maidstone MDs and five
Canterbury MDs, 1660–1720

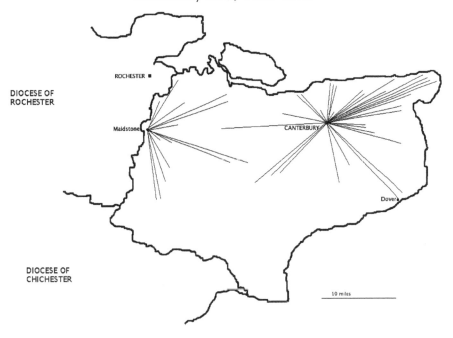

while the social range served by MDs seems to have been narrowing to the top end of the scale, their geographical range remained extensive.

The best represented medical degree-holders from medical towns outside Canterbury are John Golder of Dover, David Jones, Thomas Thorpe and Charles Nichols of Faversham, and Robert Stapley, William Belcher and Griffith Hatley of Maidstone. All seven of these men were practising in the second half of the seventeenth century, and appear in a total of ninety probate accounts. They therefore represent the most highly qualified urban physicians outside Canterbury. Notably, 29 per cent of their patients were from status groups C or D, almost twice as many as for the Canterbury MDs. But this generalisation itself masks considerable variation: in particular the exclusively high status of those served by Dr Hatley and Dr Belcher of Maidstone and Thomas Thorpe MB of Faversham. Generally the remits of physicians in these towns were smaller: 57 per cent of their clientele were from their own towns (compared to 32 per cent for the Canterbury MDs) but this too masks exceptions, for what is interesting about this comparison is how Maidstone MDs dominated the western half of the diocese in a similar way to that in which Canterbury MDs dominated the eastern half, and yet Dr Golder in Dover and Dr Jones and Dr Nichols in Faversham hardly left their own doorsteps, and as many as half of Thomas Thorpe's high-status patients

Table 54
Relative accessibility of all East Kent physicians and surgeons named in the probate accounts

	1570–1649	1660–1720
Canterbury	0.36	0.47
Major medical towns	0.38	0.54
Lesser medical towns	0.50	0.72
Rural parishes	0.10	0.55
Generally	0.34	0.55

Note: Relative accessibility is the proportion of medical assistance purchased on behalf of lower status patients relative to higher status patients. Parity would by 1.0.

Table 55
Relative accessibility of diocesan-licensed surgeons and diocesan-licensed physicians

	1570–1649		1660–1720	
	Surgery	Physic	Surgery	Physic
Canterbury	0.41	–	0.71	–
Major medical towns	0.69	0.52	0.50	0.67
Lesser medical towns	0.56	–	0.61	–
Rural parishes	0.04	0.20	0.23	0.57
Generally	0.42	0.45	0.61	0.66

Note: Relative accessibility is the proportion of medical assistance purchased on behalf of lower status patients relative to higher status patients. Parity would by 1.0.

were from his hometown (Faversham). Although the numbers are small, it would appear that medical degree-holders in the two most important towns in the later seventeenth century were exclusive, high-status practitioners who served the wealthy and the well-connected throughout the diocese; those in the smaller medical towns served local communities and were less exclusive.

Although several medical degree-holders were resident in parishes outside the medical towns, these were normally only just outside, in suburban parishes (for example, Otham, just outside Maidstone). There is no evidence of any of these men actually practising in these places. Of the very few who are known to have been resident in lesser medical towns and rural parishes, the probate accounts clearly mention only two as practising: John Hinton of Linton (d. 1698) and Isaac Warquin of New Romney. Dr Hinton is noted as serving two Status A patients in parishes a short distance from Linton (Chart Sutton and Sutton Valence); Dr Warquin falls more clearly into the pattern observable for practitioners in Dover and Faversham, treating three Status C patients as well as three Status A patients, all from the immediate vicinity, no further away than Ivychurch (the adjacent parish) and Dymchurch (three miles away).

The exclusivity of diocesan licentiates

The section above suggested a means by which the relative accessibility of a type of practitioner to lower status patients could be measured. Although it is relatively crude since it relates only to named practitioners and depends on the average higher status individuals as a constant (whereas in fact the wealth of higher status individuals in the period after 1685 was accelerating rapidly), it may be used to determine the relative accessibility of any substantial group of practitioners in any wide area. This includes the degree to which lower status patients could access physicians and surgeons generally (*see* table 54).

It seems that access by lower status patients to named physicians and surgeons in all areas increased significantly over the seventeenth century. That much might have been predicted, but less predictable is the degree to which various types of practitioner were accessible to Status C, D and S patients. The accessibility of medical degree-holders, for instance, was comparable to that of all named practitioners prior to c. 1650, but after that date they became comparatively exclusive. Table 55 includes all unambiguous references to practitioners licensed for surgery only, and practitioners licensed for physic only, by the diocesan authorities, excluding all those with a medical degree. (It also excludes all archiepiscopal licentiates and practitioners licensed by the diocese to practise both physic and surgery.)

Diocesan licentiates in both arts became more accessible to lower status patients after 1660, even though the wealth gap between them and the notional higher status patient against which they are being compared was increasing considerably. Moreover in rural areas it seems to have been starting from a very low level, as far as can be judged on the basis of the few figures available for this region. Nor can this be explained simply by their greater numbers, for it is unlikely that there were significantly more licentiates in Kent in 1660–1720 than in 1570–1649. With the exclusivity of practitioners universally declining (except in the case of Canterbury medical degree-holders) the change cannot but be linked with two previously identified factors. First, that practitioners were increasingly living in more rural areas; and second, the higher proportion of urban physicians and surgeons attending patients in person and finding markets in rural parishes.

The range of physicians and surgeons

The examination of medical degree-holders noted that a very large proportion of the diocese was covered by Canterbury-based practitioners, and a similarly large proportion was covered by Maidstone-based practitioners. Was such an extensive range just a feature of the most highly qualified, or were physicians and surgeons from lesser towns regularly covering such distances?

The practices of named physicians (excluding medical degree-holders) and surgeons from two major medical towns – Sittingbourne and Ashford – have been mapped along with Hythe, a lesser medical town whose practitioners also served a high proportion of people from other communities (see figure 13). Proximity is certainly evident: most rural patients who used physicians and surgeons from one of these towns lived within four miles of it. But this may well be symptomatic of local practitioners being those best known to and most trusted by the patients. Beyond the four-mile hinterland, proximity played little part. New Romney and Lydd practitioners have not been mapped, but without doubt they included among their clientele many from the parishes of Ivychurch, Dymchurch and St Mary in the Marsh. People from these places might equally have used Hythe practitioners (especially residents of Dymchurch) and people in all three parishes used Ashford practitioners. Patients from New Romney and Ivychurch even went as far as Sittingbourne on occasion, by-passing Ashford altogether.

The three- or four-mile hinterland of each place which may be considered 'proximity' (to use Sawyer's term) was not a hard-and-fast boundary; in certain circumstances surgeons and physicians might be sought from much further afield, and in such cases proximity was not a factor influencing the choice of practitioner. Areas of coverage from each town crossed substantially, so that the area between Sittingbourne and Ashford, or between Ashford and Hythe was not a fringe but a large swathe where patients might use the services of either town, depending on their perceived needs.

The range of rural practitioners

The picture for medical towns is clear. What remains much more of a mystery is the range of rural practitioners' practices. Hitherto it has generally been accepted that rural practitioners served their own rural communities. Clergymen in particular were thought to be in the ascendancy in rural areas, exclusively serving their own flock. The preceding sections raise a question mark over this assumption since they show that before 1650 patients from their same parishes made up only 17 per cent of the clients of named rural practitioners, and that these were moreover very exclusive practitioners. That said, in rural areas a practitioner could receive several patients from neighbouring but not distant parishes who nevertheless count as being of a different community.

Figure 13
Area covered by physicians and surgeons based in Sittingbourne, Ashford and Hythe, c. 1590–1720

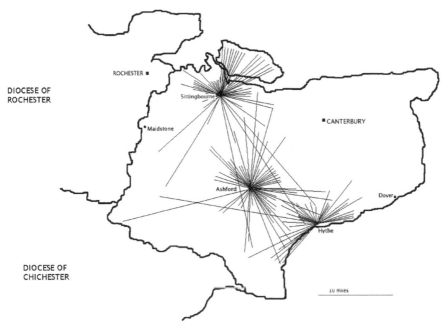

The pre-1650 rural practices in East Kent for which there is evidence are those of Walter Jones of Benenden, Alexander Devison of Staple-next-Wingham, Thomas Waterman of Pluckley, Edward Pell of Smarden, Simon Rose of Chislet and John and Thomas Smith of St Johns Thanet.[22] With the exception of the Thanet practitioners, none of these practices was restricted to adjacent parishes, and several men went much further, demonstrating as great a range as the Ashford practitioners in figure 13. Few payments were local. The pattern seems to be that rural practitioners acted in a similar fashion to high-status Canterbury practitioners, travelling long distances and showing relatively little allegiance to their hometowns. All but Thomas Waterman was licensed, and attracted high-status clients: the average wealth of Alexander Devison's five patients was £374; the average of Simon Rose's (an archiepiscopal licentiate in physic) was £478. Neither of these practitioners is recorded in the context of a lower status account.

The situation after 1660 shows little variation, only a larger number of rural practices.[23] Although more rural practitioners were serving patients from their own parishes, these practitioners still travelled long distances.

[22] These are mapped in Mortimer, 'Medical assistance', i. 235.
[23] These are mapped ibid. i. 236.

Alexander Devison's practice in Staple-next-Wingham seems to have been continued by William Spratt, based in Wingham (the next parish). The three pre-1650 practices based in Smarden, Pluckley and Biddenden seem to have shifted to Smarden and Charing, and the area to the south-east of Maidstone seems to have acquired its own practitioners. The initial local service in Thanet seems to have grown considerably in strength, to the point where the regularity of service to the local community resembles that of a small town. Sheppey may well have been following the Thanet model: dependent on medical towns in the earlier period, increasingly self-sufficient after 1660. It is noticeable, however, that the Sheppey practitioners were not licensed, and thus differ from the Thanet practitioners, who were all licensed except for Nicholas Chewney. Indeed, all the practitioners who may be associated with a particular parish – Simon Hammond of Bearsted, John Hinton of Linton, William Silvester of Sheerness, Anthony Johnson of Chilham, Thomas Meere of Marden, William Spratt of Wingham, Matthew Hartnupp of Smarden, George Brown of Smarden, James Fowtrell of Charing, John Wood of Ruckinge, George Hammon of Whitstable, Isaac Pierse, Henry Pemble and Henry Somes of Eythorne, and Ludovic Leese, John Watts, Edward Jarvis and Nicholas Chewney of St Johns Thanet – were licensed with the exceptions of those of Chewney, Pemble and Silvester. No unlicensed rural practitioners were regularly named in these accounts (unlike unlicensed urban practitioners).

Clergymen

While the reasoning underlying Sawyer's explanation of why clergymen and gentlewomen might have played 'a huge role' in the provision of medical care (which was based on a proximity definition of ten miles) is not tenable, this does not rule out the suggestion that either group may have served extensively in a medical capacity.[24] Unfortunately, in this respect, it is not possible to use probate accounts to quantify or even to illustrate the role of the clergy. Accounts record medical intervention only in those cases where payment is concerned; therefore charitable acts do not feature. It is perhaps not surprising that there are very few appearances in these documents of members of the clergy acting in a medical capacity. It is probable that clergymen felt that charging for their predominantly charitable services was incompatible with the death of a patient, especially since they would have to charge for his burial and a funeral sermon.

Nine practitioners have been identified who were also clergymen before 1650 (Henoch Clapham, Francis Fotherbie, Edmund Henshaw, Randolph Partridge, Mr Sewell, Thomas Turner, William Turner, Harimo White and

Theophilus White) and three after 1660 (Henry Nicholls, John Swan and William Stringer). Most of these practitioners are known only from their having been granted a licence or awarded a medical degree; only five appear in a probate account. Of these five, two were not licensed. The first of them was Francis Fotherbie, vicar of Linsted, who was paid in 1646 for treating a child of the deceased who was ill with 'the ricketts'; he was not actually paid for treating the deceased.[25] The other was Mr Sewell, rector of Shadoxhurst, who was paid for 'phisick for the said deceased' in 1614.[26] This entry might represent a debt as much as a payment for medical assistance: if Mr Sewell had obtained from an apothecary – or otherwise provided – medicines at a cost to himself, he may well have felt justified in passing that cost on, in spite of his patient's death. The same may be said for a third clergyman, Edmund Henshaw, vicar of Sutton Valence, a licensed physician, who was paid by a parishioner 'for physic fetched for the deceased in the time of his sickness' in 1639.[27] The remaining two clergymen noted, John Swan and Randolph Partridge, probably were not practitioners at the same time as they were clergymen. Swan was a minister of Ockenham who had taken his BA in 1639 but who was ejected for nonconformity. It is probable that this took place before he became an ecclesiastical licentiate in medicine, as he is described as 'of Hougham' in the licence. He is mentioned in an account dated 1665 as 'Doctor Swanne' when he was paid 'for phisicke by him administered unto the said deceased in the time of the sicknes whereof he died'.[28] The last man, Randolph Partridge, was consistently described in the accounts as an apothecary. He seems not to have combined this business with being the curate of Sutton by Dover but rather, like John Swan, to have performed each role sequentially. He was curate from 1619 to 1625; the twelve accounts in which he is named all date from before this period or after it. In fact he obtained his licence to practise physic in the year after he ceased to be curate, perhaps after encountering religious hostility.[29] It appears that his return to a medical career, properly licensed, was a path subsequent to his curacy, and one which he continued until emigrating in 1637. The lack of any evidence for his charging while acting as curate means that there is very little evidence – just the two possible cases concerning Sewell and Henshaw – of any serving clergyman charging the family of a dying patient for medical assistance.

This begs the question: to what extent did the clergy provide medical help to the seriously ill and dying in East Kent? The simple answer is that there is no sure way of knowing. However, certain points are worth noting.

25 PRC 1/7/86.
26 PRC 2/18/27.
27 PRC 1/2/69.
28 PRC 1/10/68. He may also have been the 'Doctor Swan' paid for 'phisick' given to a wealthy Appledore man in 1690: PRC 19/4/119.
29 See his entry in J. Venn, *Alumni cantabrigienses*, pt I, Cambridge 1922–7.

The first is that there were very few clergymen licensed to practise medicine. This must be considered curious in a diocese where all the indicators are that there was a stricter adherence to the ecclesiastical licensing laws than elsewhere, with more than 30 per cent of all known practitioners being licensed, even in the period 1570–1610 (for which licensing records are scarce). If the six clergy licensed between 1608 and 1635 represent 30 per cent of all the clergymen who regularly practised medicine in the diocese, then the total number would have been just twenty, or 10 per cent of the probable total number of practitioners working in the diocese. It is likely that some other practitioners were clergymen who did not seek a medical licence, but if there were many of these, why did they not take out a licence when so many laymen did? One answer to this question might be that they were working on a very part-time basis. Another might be that they attended only minor cases, perhaps restricting their medical interventions to children and mild illnesses. However, probably the most likely answer is that there were so many medical practitioners in the diocese – at least one practitioner for every 400 people – that the medical role of the clergy was not as important as Sawyer suggests. This must certainly be the case in respect of the seriously ill. After 1660, when medical strategies to cope with serious and fatal illnesses were becoming universal, and licensing seems to have been a system as scrupulously adhered to as before, just three clergymen are known to have held a medical licence: the aforesaid John Swan, William Stringer (from the diocese) in 1673 and Henry Nicholls (from the College of Physicians) in 1684.

A further reason to doubt that the clergy were playing a major medical role towards the seriously ill and dying in East Kent lies in the fact that only two serving clergymen appear in these accounts as supplying physic. Although it is likely that clergymen waived their fees for treating the dying, this does not explain why so few were paid for supplying physic or medicines (only two certain cases out of more than 4,000). The average prices of medical substances noted in these accounts were not inconsiderable: rarely were payments for medicines less than 5s., whether from doctors, apothecaries or physicians. Even if clergymen waived any fees they might have charged for attendance on the dying, not all could have afforded in every case to waive the costs of obtaining the medicines they supplied. Nor can it credibly be argued that in all but two cases the clergy were acting as non-dispensing physicians, acting only in an advisory capacity, when it has been shown that physicians frequently dispensed medicine themselves in rural areas. It has to be concluded that, in East Kent, clergymen were not supplying medicines to the seriously ill and dying in any significant quantities. It follows that, while it is not possible to determine the level of medical help offered by them overall, it is very unlikely that in this diocese they regularly took a part in treating the dying, and one must seriously question whether the 'huge role' which Sawyer claims for them in Buckinghamshire in the early seventeenth century is applicable in East Kent.

Female practitioners

In his discussion of proximity, Sawyer argued that gentlewomen as well as clergymen were important in the provision of rural medical assistance.[30] As very few women have been mentioned so far, it might be considered that females did not have a major part in the medical care (as opposed to nursing care) of the dying. However, the role of women as evidenced in these accounts is a complicated matter. The problem lies in occupational designations: females hardly feature at all in the thousands of references to physicians and surgeons. There is just one reference in the Kent accounts to 'a woman physician' and one reference to 'two women Chirurgions'.[31] Women are recorded as taking part in healing processes and supplying medicines but they were not normally assigned medical identities.

This presents a very different situation to that of examining male medical roles. With men there is a dichotomy between looking at the practitioner from the perspective of his occupational identity and from his patients' perspective in describing his service. With women there is no such dichotomy, owing to the near-complete absence of female medical identities. The problem is rather the opposite: trying to distinguish whether women who merely assisted as part of a local labour force had medical identities of their own which were not expressed overtly in the accounts. In other words, is it possible to distinguish a significant branch of female medical assistance distinct from palliative care?

To answer this, it is first necessary to consider all the medical payments which were made exclusively to women (setting aside payments such as 'Paid to the Doctor and a woman for physic and attendance' as ambiguous). In terms of service rendered, this includes payments to women for surgery, for provision of physic, for advice and for 'curing' (or applying a specific remedy). It might also include some payments for 'attending' or 'tending' and 'keeping', but since payments for these services are normally indistinguishable from palliative care, they are dealt with in chapter 5.

There are only two unambiguous references to a woman being paid for giving medical advice. The first is a payment of 32s. in an account dated 1635 on behalf of a Status D man from Postling 'to one Mrs Wright of or about Canterbury for phisick by her ministred to the said testator in the time of his sicknes and for her advise thereabouts and her paynes and charges in coming and horsehire in fetching her twise from Canterbury to Postling to doo the same'.[32] The second is Mrs Jacob of Canterbury, who was almost certainly a member of the very extensive family of practitioners based in that city. In 1639 10s. was paid on behalf of a Status B man, William Maxted,

---

[30] On the subject of gentlewomen practitioners see also Nagy, *Popular medicine*, 54–78.
[31] PRC 1/8/2, PRC 2/24/34, dated 1648 and 1624 respectively.
[32] PRC 2/33/12.

'to Mrs Jacob for her directions in physic'.[33] This Mrs Jacob was probably the same as the Mrs Jacob mentioned in a 1649 account giving advice in conjunction with her son, 14s. being paid on behalf of a Status A Canterbury man, 'to Mrs Jacob and her son for their advice and counsell and for physick had of them in the time of the said deceased's last sickness whereof he died'.[34] These are the only references to women giving medical 'advice' to the dying and in view of the probable relationship of one of them to a dynasty of well-qualified city apothecaries and physicians, it is difficult to regard the latter as one of the well-meaning rural gentlewomen to whom Sawyer was referring.

There are a further forty-three references to women in connection with a medical function.[35] These do not all suggest the application of female medical skill. A payment in 1637 to John Brent's maid and one in 1665 to Joanne Grigges 'the deceaseds daughter' are both for fetching physic, and amounted to no more medical intervention than travelling into a town to purchase certain medicines. Entries such as 'paid for physic and for two women for watching with the deceased' give no certain indication that the women were employed in anything other than a palliative role, or that there is any connection between them and the purchase of physic. A third ambiguous entry is to be found in an account dated 1662, 'paid to Mrs Fearne for looking to and attendance upon the said deceased'. Whether cases of 'looking to' and 'attendance' relate to medical or merely palliative care cannot be judged. Even if it is possible in some instances to ascertain whether this form of words was intended to reflect a medical or palliative role, it is not possible to do so over such a large sweep of time.

Six of the female practitioner entries directly relate to the medical care of children of the deceased, and one to an apprentice. This compares with a total of forty-eight male practitioners recorded in payments for medical assistance to children of the deceased. Female practitioners might be said to have provided about 13 per cent of the paid medical care to children in these accounts (excluding wet-nursing and children taken ill due to multiple infections spreading through the house). This is strikingly in excess of the degree to which women are recorded unambiguously in medical roles treating dying adults. It is furthermore in accord with an opinion expressed by Sir Ralph Verney, that old women 'by experience know better than any physician how to treat infants'.[36] Six of these seven payments were for healing the legs of a child, whether due to injury (as in one case) or 'soreness'. The seventh is specifically for 'curing the head' of a girl. It is interesting that this pattern of

---

[33] PRC 1/3/14.
[34] PRC 1/8/36.
[35] These are given in full in Mortimer, 'Medical assistance', ii. 88–91.
[36] A. Clark (ed. and intro. A. L. Erickson), *Working life of women in the seventeenth century*, London 1992, 258.

descriptions of treating specific, limited ailments is repeated for adults. Of the remaining payments to female practitioners, one is for treating gravel (1640 Hythe West, 'abroke'), two are for general 'sores' (1641 Dymchurch, 1682 Faversham), four were for 'sore legs' (1624 Teynham, 1634 Fordwich, 1641 New Romney, 1722 Herne), five were for 'sore throats' (1628 Sandwich, 1634 Biddenden, 1637 Canterbury, 1639 Canterbury, 1649 Canterbury) and one last one was for treating a mouth complaint (1675 Canterbury). While it would be wrong to assume that such ailments were of a slight nature, the very limited and precise description of the disease differentiates these payments from the vast majority, and suggests that they were not perceived to be causes of death. Indeed, several state that the female practitioners were paid for 'healing' and 'curing' these cases; none of them is given the common addendum 'in the time of the sickness whereof he died'.

In total, of the forty-three payments to female practitioners, two were for nothing more than fetching medicines, seven were for tending children, thirteen were for treating limited, minor ailments, and twenty-one were for surgery and providing physic to the deceased. In addition to the two women who were described as offering advice, it would appear that only two dozen women were undoubtedly employed in medical roles helping the dying, compared to 1,756 males. So substantial a male dominance in the context of the seriously ill and dying clearly raises a number of questions about medical care in the last days of life, especially as such lives usually ended in the home. Thus these figures, which suggest that women were responsible for less than 2 per cent of the paid medical assistance to the dying in the long seventeenth century, require further comment.

For a start the ambiguity of the language must be borne in mind: by excluding words such as 'attended' and 'tending' and 'looking to' the possibility is dismissed that women from outside the home were obtaining medicines and administering them on their own initiative, thereby acting in a paid medical capacity. Since there are more than a thousand references to women 'attending', 'tending' or 'looking to', this problem cannot easily be ignored. Secondly, the bias of the courts against being seen to approve payments for medical services to women who were unlicensed (no female licentiates in the diocese of Canterbury have as yet been identified) must be considered. It is probable that very few women even attempted to break the barrier of occupational prejudice to obtain a diocesan licence to practise medicine or surgery.[37] Thus it is possible that where accounts have entries such as 'paid for physic', the roles of nurses and local attendants in prescribing and

---

[37] The diocese of Exeter, in which it seems that only one medical or surgical licence and only about ten midwifery licences were granted to women, has very few applications for either medical or midwifery licences. It would appear that the reason that they were not granted was predominantly that women did not apply for them: Mortimer, 'Diocesan licensing', 52.

providing medicines were being masked by the language of an economic transaction. In addition, it was to the accountant's advantage to cloak female medical roles in this way, or to dress them down as 'attending' or 'fetching physic', in order to lessen the chances of being called into question by the court. Female 'attendants' might have performed much the same role as a male 'physician' on occasion but to suggest that they did so to a church court would have shown scant regard for convention. Thus it is not surprising that there is only one reference to a female 'physician'; the occupational paradigm in East Kent was exclusively male.

What may be concluded is that, while formally acknowledged medical assistance to the seriously ill and dying was almost entirely provided by male practitioners, there was a significant reserve of informal female knowledge and experience which could be drawn upon by the dying and their carers. The analogy is to a wide but shallow pool of knowledge as opposed to the deeper wells of formal medical training. Women with a smattering of medical knowledge were not normally regarded as practitioners, and indeed most were not medical practitioners in an occupational sense. But there were many of them and in certain contexts they might be considered to have sufficient experience and skill in a speciality to have a popular reputation. In such cases it was justifiable for people to seek out these women and to pay for their services. On the basis of the probate account evidence it might be suggested that the key areas where women could acquire and gain a reputation as specialists included skin, mouth and throat disorders, children's problems, and 'sore' and injured limbs. Of course, these are in addition to childbirth, the one arena in which women managed to acquire formal recognition of their services.

The analogy of a shallow pool of widespread general medical knowledge with deeper areas where some women had acquired specific skills, complementing the men who plumbed the depths of formal medical training, is supported by further examination of the records of female practitioners. First, there was no collapse of payments to women in the later seventeenth century, the period when male medical practitioners' services were very widely used, which we would perhaps have been expected had there been a degree of competition, or had women's skills been amateurish by comparison with male medical knowledge. Equally important, several of these women carry reflections of higher status: Mrs Forte (1599), Mrs Clerk (1629), Mrs Wright (1635) Mrs Aldersley (1638) and Mrs Jacob (1639, 1649), Mrs Fearne (1662), Mrs Symon (1663), Mrs Bartlett (1674, twice), Mrs Robbins (1681), Mrs Nowell (1682), Mrs Nicholls (1684) and Mrs Coveny (1688). Thus about a third of female practitioners were noted as 'Mrs', a status equivalent to the 'Mr' assigned to the majority of male practitioners by about 1625. If instances are included of other women with the pretitle 'Mrs or Mistress' who are recorded as 'attending' or 'looking to' the deceased, the names of Mrs Swift (1620), Mrs Lewkner 'wyef of Alexander Lewkner' (1623), Mrs Jarvis (1628), 'Mrs Pulley the vicars wife of Throwley' (1637),

Mrs Nightingale (1677) and Mrs Wilson (1700) can be added.[38] Given the likely propensity for women to concentrate on children's diseases and non-fatal and minor ailments, including sore legs, throats and mouths (which are only rarely noted in these accounts), and given the probability that many gentlewomen did not charge for their services, especially when their patient died, there can be little doubt that these few references indicate that women of respectability continued to play an occasional medical role throughout the seventeenth century, supplementing the more regularly employed male practitioners quantified in chapter 3.

This finding would appear to support Sawyer's argument about gentle-women being required to perform a medical role in the absence of a general practitioner. However, when looking at the discrepancy between some patients' and practitioners' parishes, a different picture emerges. Widow Pye of Faversham, for instance, was sought out for her surgery wares by a patient from Harty, on the Isle of Sheppey. The services of Mrs Clerk of Canterbury were obtained on behalf of a Whitstable patient, six miles away. Mrs Wright of Canterbury was sought by a patient from Postling, more than ten miles away. Goodwife Franchle, the Hythe woman 'who professeth much skill in surgery', attended a patient in the parish of Dymchurch, between two and four miles away. Susanna Butler of Tenterden was paid for providing physic to a Woodchurch patient, at four miles distance. In none of these cases is there any evidence that the deceased died away from home and that these were charitable gentlewomen who happened to be near at hand. On the whole it appears that they were not local gentlefolk kindly assisting the poor and needy in their own parish but women who had acquired a speciality and who were being sought out by patients in the same way as such patients might seek out a male practitioner or informally trained medical functionary, like a bonesetter. It is probably no coincidence that all five of these women who dealt with patients from further afield were based in medical towns.

Distances travelled and specific services described may be counted as evidence that a number of women were providing specialist medical services as a complement to the general occupationally defined services offered by men. Another telling sign that the women recorded in these accounts were not all gentlewomen acting out of charity may be taken from the range of prices paid for medical help. Here may be seen the contrast between the 'wide shallow pool of general medical knowledge' and the specialist helpers. Those women who were described as 'chirurgions', or performing acts of 'surgery' tended to receive significant remuneration. The 'two women Chirurgions or skillfull women' who undertook to cure a running sore in 1624 were paid 60s.; Mrs Forte was paid 19s. for her surgery in 1599; Goodwife

[38] PRC 2/21/55, PRC 20/6/312, PRC 20/8/33, PRC 2/34/127, PRC 2/37/162, PRC 19/5/66.

Franchle was rewarded with 20s. for her surgery; and the female physician of Hollingbourne also received the sum of 20s.. What is significant is that some of the amounts paid for curing sore limbs were compatible with these fees. Thus what might be described as 'women's specialities' such as dealing with sore limbs can be seen to have deserved remuneration on the same scale as females practising 'surgery' and this in turn, through the language of medical occupations, hints at the comparability of some female and male medical practices. Not all female activities were highly remunerated, and the 'wide shallow pool' can perhaps be seen in the small payments paid to local women for minor cures, such as the 1s. 6d. paid to Goodwife Foxe for attending on a sore throat, or the 3s. paid to Elizabeth Wiggins or Higgins for tending to a sore leg. Finally, it is noticeable that the majority of patients employing women after 1660 were from high-status groups, whereas those employing women before 1650 were from lower status groups. The discrepancy is distinctly in excess of the bias of the sample. As medical strategies for coping with serious diseases became almost ubiquitous in the latter part of the seventeenth century, women's medical services did not get pushed down the social scale. This is further evidence that female practitioners, in certain cases, were sought after by those who could have chosen to employ male practitioners, if they had wanted to.

Arguably the most important aspect of this chapter has been the importance of the situation and scope of medical practices, and their ability to cover the whole diocese. The evidence points clearly to occupationally defined medical practitioners increasingly servicing rural parishes over the course of the seventeenth century. Although there are some exceptions, such as the town of Dover, practitioners in the major medical towns were largely catering to a widening market, the lesser medical towns were emerging as important centres with respect to their own locales and rural areas were beginning to see medicine provided by local practitioners on a regular basis.

A structured periodic model for the provision of medicine in East Kent might thus be proposed. The whole period after 1600 was one of long-term uninterrupted growth in the provision of medical services in the face of severe illness and injury, but various decades display differing characteristics which might clarify the development patterns of medical services. Three phases may be distinguished. The first is a period of very modest growth, characterised by a low level of occupationally-defined medical provision throughout the diocese, especially in rural areas. In this period practitioners were almost all situated in medical towns; hence this phase might be termed 'urban-centred'. More than half the practitioners' business involved their fellow townsmen. Outside those towns even the relatively wealthy and well-connected did not frequently obtain practitioners' assistance. It is possible that elements of the rural clergy assisted in rural areas medically, on an unpaid basis, although not in respect of the provision of expensive medicines. There was a distinct urban bias to occupational medical assistance to the dying: location close to or within a town remained a more significant medical advantage than wealth or status in obtaining medical help.

The urban-centred period shades into a second, which might be termed 'urban-distributed'. It is characterised by a much greater – and increasing – propensity for both urban and rural patients to obtain medical help but for the supply of medical assistance to remain largely in the hands of urban-based practitioners. Increasing rural demand was communicated via messengers, servants or family members sent into the medical towns, either to buy medicines or to solicit the attendance of a practitioner. This period may be said roughly to date from about 1615 in the cases of the highest status groups and from about 1635 in the cases of the lowest status groups represented in these accounts.

The second period shades into a third, 'rural-development' phase, characterised by a significant body of rural medical help being provided by a local or nearby rural source, in addition to the continued provision of medical supplies and practitioners from towns. In East Kent this transition may perhaps have started in the 1670s and gathered speed in the 1680s and 1690s. The result was that by the early eighteenth century, rural areas such as Thanet were able to make use of medical services more frequently than Canterbury and other large medical towns, having a local practitioner base as well as access to the city, six to ten miles away. Although urban areas remained pre-eminent in the supply of medical services, their hegemony was no longer absolute.

The most obvious consequence of these developments is the decline in the proportion of urban practitioners' markets represented by urban populations, the extreme being from 57 per cent to 35 per cent for Canterbury practitioners over the seventeenth century. Other features include the decline in exclusivity for most types of practitioners over the period, with the exception of the increasing exclusivity of the most highly qualified in the last phase, the increasing proportions of named practitioners who held some form of qualification and the decreasing consistency of practitioner nomenclature. From the patients' point of view, practitioners were becoming increasingly homogenised as 'doctors', regardless of the nature of their qualifications. It could even be suggested that by 1700 most officially recognised practitioners were considered to be practitioners of general medicine by large portions of the population, with the exceptions of urban apothecaries and those surgeons who were widely known specifically to have concentrated on their surgical skills.

This provides a new framework for understanding the emergence of the general practitioner in East Kent. That only one specific reference possibly relates to an apothecary working from a rural location very strongly suggests that the designation 'apothecary' in this period was popularly considered in East Kent to be an exclusively urban one. This runs contrary to the traditional belief that in England the surgeon-apothecary was the forerunner of the general practitioner and the occupational designation which was to be associated with bringing medicine into rural areas. In East Kent rural patients described the men who treated them in person as doctors, surgeons and physicians, not 'surgeon-apothecaries'. These men may well have been performing exactly the same tasks as the surgeon-apothecary – they were certainly supplying drugs as well as giving advice – but the East Kent accountants made a clear distinction between the urban apothecary and the provincial physician, and this was the case long before 1700. It would be more accurate to say that, in East Kent, the role associated with the provincial physician or doctor, which developed in the later seventeenth century, was much the same as that associated later with the general practitioner, and this was underpinned by a number of types of qualification, the most common of which was the licence to practise surgery. What is important to realise is that, in most medical towns, one man could perform both roles – that of urban apothecary and that of provincial physician – at the same time, although in Canterbury most apothecaries stuck to the former.

Comparability

It is difficult to test the development of medical services in other dioceses. Not only do many fewer documents survive, but fewer of them record medical intervention due to the 'filtrations' discussed in chapter 2, and still fewer name the practitioner paid. Only a handful gives details of both the practitioner's hometown and his occupational designation. Furthermore, the information available regarding diocesan licensing is poor by comparison with that for the diocese of Canterbury. Some checks are nevertheless possible.

Assuming, for the sake of argument, that apothecaries in Berkshire were largely or exclusively based in medical towns, as in East Kent, of the twenty Berkshire payments to apothecaries dated 1592–1641, fourteen were made on behalf of patients in major medical towns (70 per cent), whereas nine of the thirty-two accounts dated 1663–92 were for residents of medical towns (28 per cent).[39] This drop is in no way attributable to shifts in the sample as the proportion of accounts relating to residents of medical towns across the period decreases only marginally.[40] Thus, wherever the Berkshire apothecaries were based, their market was shifting, like in East Kent, from one dominated by residents of medical towns to one inclusive of many rural parishes.

---

[39] The comparable figures for West Sussex are 3/13 (earlier period) and 0/5 (later period) and for Wiltshire 2/5 (earlier period) and 12/26 (later period).
[40] This is measured across the period 1590–1649 compared to 1660–99. The figures for Berkshire are 961/1250 (77%) accounts outside medical towns in 1590–1649 and 363/462 (79%) in 1660–99. The figures for West Sussex are 657/805 (82%) accounts outside medical towns in 1590–1649 and 301/368 (82%) in 1660–99.

The problem is that this conclusion is based on just fifty-two accounts: too few to be convincing. What is required is a broader view of medical interventions in the central southern counties. Assuming that a model is being tested which depends on a balance between medical consumption in towns and rural areas, if rural patients were receiving a greater proportion of the total medical assistance available, then the proportion represented by urban patients must have been decreasing, and the region must either have been experiencing an urban-distributed phase (if the medical assistance was being provided by urban practitioners) or a rural-development one (if a significant number of rural medical practitioners was involved). The urban/hinterland ratio for higher status patients in East Kent decreased from 1.7 in 1600–49 to 1.3 in 1660–89. For the lower status groups the ratio dropped from 1.85 to 1.3. These figures may be directly compared with other counties to see what level of medical care was obtained by rural patients. If Berkshire and West Sussex were, like Kent, seeing more medical care purchased on behalf of rural patients, then there should be a trend towards convergence similar to that in East Kent.

Berkshire and West Sussex demonstrate strikingly different development patterns. In Berkshire, the urban: hinterland ratio of the higher status groups hardly alters over the century, remaining at about 1.1–1.25. The same can be said for the higher status groups in West Sussex, which remained at about 1.6–1.7. The urban/hinterland ratio for the lower status groups in both counties was around 2.8–2.9 in the earlier period, and, as far as can be ascertained, was just as high in West Sussex at the end of the century. It is with regard to the rural lower status groups in Berkshire that signs of change can be perceived. In Berkshire, like East Kent, there was an increasing tendency to provide medical relief for seriously ill rural lower status patients. It would appear that Sussex did not follow this trend at the same time.

With regard to practitioner descriptions, it was noted that in East Kent these were becoming much looser after 1660. This change was considered indicative of practitioners increasingly being considered 'general', even where specifically licensed to perform only surgery. Although it is not possible to check this in the same way for Berkshire and West Sussex, the most obvious feature of the less consistent nomenclature was the great increase in references to 'doctors'. This is found paralleled closely in both West Sussex and Berkshire. In East Kent the frequency with which the word was used rose from 9 per cent (1570–1649) to 29 per cent (1660–1720) for higher status patients and from 6 per cent to 22 per cent for lower status. The comparable rise in Berkshire was from 0 (1590–1649) to 23 per cent (1660–89) for higher status patients, and from 1 per cent to 21 per cent for lower status. The increases in West Sussex were from 4 per cent to 29 per cent (higher status) and 4 per cent to 45 per cent (lower status).[41]

---

[41] Mortimer, 'Medical assistance', i. 254.

A similar increase is to be noted in the use of the description 'apothecary' in Berkshire. In East Kent, where this is an exclusively urban designation, the proportion of practitioners so called declined from 14 per cent to 8 per cent for higher status groups and from 11 per cent to 6 per cent for lower status; and a similar drop is noticeable in Sussex. But in Berkshire such descriptions increased from 17 per cent to 38 per cent for the higher status and from 17 per cent to 34 per cent for lower status groups. At the same time in Berkshire there are indications that 'apothecaries' might attend the sick and dying: one clear reference being 'payd to Mr Sellwood the apothecary [of Abingdon] for physick & his attendance' on a Status B patient at Long Wittenham in Berkshire in 1687.[42] It may well be that in Mr Sellwood we can see the importance of the 'surgeon-apothecaries' reflected in this high number of references to 'apothecaries', and confirmation that they were attending like the 'doctors' so frequently mentioned in East Kent and West Sussex. The only Sussex equivalent to Mr Sellwood is 'paid Mr Vavsour for coming to him' referring to the Chichester practitioner Thomas Vavasour, who travelled to Boxgrove to attend a Status C patient in 1676.[43] Mr Vavasour was described in other accounts as 'apothecary', 'physician' and 'doctor'. He was a licentiate in medicine, and thus had a number of medical roles.

In Berkshire the increase in medical assistance is most noticeable in the case of lower status groups in rural areas. Logically, if rural lower status groups were increasing their medical assistance faster than any other group, and if this increase was not due to the greater accessibility of lower status groups to physicians and surgeons generally, it probably was due to their geographical position. It seems reasonable to suggest that people living in rural or hinterland areas of Berkshire purchased medicine and advice with a greater frequency after about 1640–60, but that the status threshold as to who might record a medical payment dropped. This would mean that a new market was opening up to Berkshire practitioners, that of the less well-off rural patient. The group most probably responsible for the 'new markets' was styled 'apothecaries', but whether apothecaries in Berkshire were associated exclusively with medical towns, as they were in East Kent, cannot easily be established.[44] There is no evidence that Berkshire practitioners were becoming increasingly rural, and with only one unambiguous reference to a Berkshire apothecary attending the sick, it must be assumed that most of these medical interventions were characterised by representatives of the seriously ill and dying patients purchasing medicines or 'cures' from practitioners based in towns.

In West Sussex there was a similar take-up of medical strategies around the time of the Interregnum whereby urban as well as rural higher status groups doubled their use of medicine, and urban and rural lower status groups

[42] BRO, D/A1/189/19C.
[43] WSRO, EpI/33/1676/17.
[44] Nine home towns can be identified for Berkshire apothecaries: all are medical towns.

trebled theirs. Rural markets in West Sussex were also opening up to practitioners, but in this case they were more frequently styled 'doctors' than
'apothecaries'. Significantly, in West Sussex it was not just in rural areas that
new markets were being found, for it would appear that the relative accessibility of medical care increased generally (from 0.55 to 0.95, almost parity),
and the contemporary increase in urban areas suggests that improvements in
communications were not the sole or even the principal means of change.

Such a reading of the evidence suggests that Berkshire and Sussex
broadly followed East Kent in shifting from an urban-centred to an urban-
distributed phase of medical development. This situation does not seem to
have prevailed in neighbouring Wiltshire, where there is no indication that
an urban-centred phase gave way to an urban-distributed one. In fact the
rural lower status groups in Wiltshire do not seem to have benefited at all.
The use of 'doctors' and apothecaries remained largely a high-status affair.
Whereas West Sussex lower status groups had easy access to medical practitioners after 1660, and Berkshire lower status groups had better access than
previously, the less well-off in Wiltshire did not, and those who did obtain
their services lived in towns. This not only suggests a more socially exclusive
urban-distributed phase, it raises the question of the extent to which medical
assistance was obtained freely on behalf of this group. For the tricky subject
of the clergy, there is even less evidence than for East Kent. All that can
be said is that the clergy exhibit the same elusiveness: there are no clear
payments to clergymen for medical assistance in any of these counties, nor
for medical provision, and only one payment for therapeutic accommodation
while a rector's wife attended to a child's sore leg.

Finally there is the question of female assistance. As with East Kent,
payments to women for medical assistance are very few and far between, and
mostly limited to carrying out cures on children or skin and throat ailments
of the deceased. In Berkshire there is a single unambiguous reference: 'to Mrs
Smith for physicke' on behalf of a Welford patient in 1668.[45] In Wiltshire
there are two: 'Imprimis paid Jane Bond for giving of glisters' on behalf of
a Chippenham patient in 1679[46] and 'to one Mistress White of Hanly for
curinge a scaldinge of his handes and armes' on behalf of a Fovant patient
in 1632.[47] In West Sussex there are seven payments relating to women
and medical assistance. One of these is 'to Mrs Peachey for medicines &
physick for the deceased in his sickness' (Mrs Peachey probably being the
wife of Mr Peachey, the surgeon). [48] Three are more obviously for female
medical involvement: 'payd to Mrs Chalcroft for iourneys & Physicke for the
deceased in the time of his sicknes' (Rustington, 1682),[49] 'paid the Widdow

45 BRO, D/A1/120/153D.
46 WRO, P3/C/332.
47 WRO, P2/F/153.
48 WSRO, EpI/33/1682/11.
49 WSRO, EpI/33/1682/36.

French for curinge of Jane Parsons' (Wiston, 1670, where Jane was the wife of the deceased who also died, despite the 'curinge'),[50] and 'paid to Mrs Elizabeth Rose for physicke & surgery in the time of the lameness & sicknesse of the deceased' (Aldingbourne, 1682).[51] Notably, all of these payments are post-1660, and thus do not conform with Sawyer's theory of gentlewomen helping patients in medically desolate rural areas; rather they are contemporary with the significant expansion in medical assistance and are in accord with the payments to similar women in East Kent at this time. The last three payments which relate to female medical help are all pre-1650: 'given Mrs Bond for her payns taken abowt the Cure of the said henrie Strudweeke in glasses & bottles to the value of 10s' (Kirdford, 1612),[52] 'to goodman Danyell of West Grinsted for going to the Countess of [Elye?] for phisicke' (Shipley, 1631),[53] and to the rector of Petworth in 1600 for looking after 'one of the children of the said John Hamon during which time Mrs Borde the wife of the said Dr Borde had him in care for the heale[ing] of his sore legg'.[54] The last of these is reminiscent of Sawyer's role for rural clergy and gentlewomen, but it was in Petworth, one of the medical towns, and not a rural area. As for the Countess of Ely, there was no such title in 1631, and this remains somewhat mysterious; it perhaps related to the sign of an inn. The important point is that, if women could be mentioned in all these dioceses as providing medical care, why were they recorded so infrequently unless they were not providing a paid medical service? And why were so many payments made on behalf of children or for damaged legs, skin etc? The extent to which women did attend the seriously ill and dying in a medical capacity, whether as lay healers or occupational practitioners has to be questioned; as does the degree to which their role (medical or otherwise) was interpreted purely within the parameters of palliative care.

[50] WSRO, EpI/33/1670/25.
[51] WSRO, EpI/33/1682/40.
[52] WSRO, EpI/33/1612/10.
[53] WSRO, EpI/33/1631/33.
[54] WSRO, EpI/33/1600/2.

5

The Nature and Availability of Nursing Care

'In England and on the continent the secular nurse was illiterate, heavy-handed, venal and over-worked. She divided her time between housework, laundry, scrubbing and a pretence at nursing of the most rough and ready kind. She seldom refused a fee and often demanded it. Strong drink was her weakness, and often her refuge from the drudgery of her life. She was not often young, but was usually a middle-aged woman, often a powerful virago … Because of her type the average family of those days [eighteenth century] dreaded and avoided the hired nurse and dosed themselves with home-made medicines.'[1]

We have come a long way since the above lines were written. We no longer regard nurses as often drunk, nor do we regard their being middle-aged as 'a bad thing', and we do not presume that it was only because the 'hired nurse' was so feared that households armed themselves with recipes from medical do-it-yourself books. We accept the need for many of them to be paid. We understand the context of Cruikshank's famous drawing of an ugly nurse, with her lantern and urine flask, much more in the humour in which it was drawn – as a parody of extremes – and not as an attempt accurately to portray those who cared for the sick. But we still make assumptions about nursing. In particular, we still tend to assume (on the whole) that nurses were female.[2] There is an assumption, perhaps growing among historians of female labour, that nursing was a significant income-generating occupation for women.[3] There is also a refusal to see the origins of modern nursing as extending back into the period under study.[4] At the same time there is a declared point of view that, prior to the late seventeenth century, women provided the bulk of everyday healing care.[5] Since people died regularly, on a weekly basis in many parishes if not a daily one, and given the findings of the previous chap-

---

1   L. Dock and I. Stewart, *A short history of nursing from the earliest times to the present day*, 4th edn, New York 1938, 98.
2   With regard to nursing the dying see S. Mendelson and P. Crawford, *Women in early modern England*, Oxford 1998, and Erickson, in the introduction to Clark, *Working life of women*, p. xxxiii. With regard to nursing generally see B. Abel-Smith, *A history of the nursing profession*, London 1960, where nursing is associated exclusively with women.
3   See P. Sharpe, *Women's work: the English experience, 1650–1914*, London 1998.
4   Several modern studies date the origin of nursing even later than Abel-Smith (who dated it to c. 1800), usually to the mid-nineteenth century. C. Maggs, *The origins of general nursing*, London 1983, concentrates upon an even later period, 1881–1914.
5   M. Versluysen, 'Old wives' tales? Women healers in English history', in C. Davies (ed.), *Rewriting nursing history*, London 1980, 175–99.

ters, we have to wonder whether this too is not a presumption, since many seriously ill people adopted medical strategies. Although progress has been made since the quotation that headed this chapter was written, substantially more enlightenment cannot be claimed.

Defining nursing

Margaret Pelling's essay, 'Nurses and nursekeepers', is pivotal in the historiography of the subject. Pelling moves away from a static viewpoint or definition and expresses a concept of nursing which is multi-dimensional, incorporating gender roles, social obligations, economic strategies, literary stereotypes and social exclusion. Her starting point is the 'joint orientation' approach to women's work put forward by Harriet Bradley.[6] Rather than presenting women as a 'reserve army of labour' and a predominantly unskilled labour force, Pelling views them as concerned with economic as well as family objectives, in her words 'productive' as well as 'reproductive' obligations. She argues that to regard women as a pool of unskilled labour is to mistake the lack of occupational identity reflected in the records for a lack of designated function. In her vision of the labour force, seventeenth-century women took on a variety of roles in much the same way as men, often part-time, often simultaneously multi-tasking, but lacking the occupational identity assigned to men. This allows her to stress the areas of overlap in women's (and men's) caring roles: the medical aspects which were a subset of acting as a nurse, and the nursing roles which were a subset of acting in a medical capacity, and the medical and nursing subsets of simply being present and concerned for the patient. The logical progression of this approach is to define sick-nursing as several functions which in theory anyone could do (in the same way that anyone could build a house in theory), but which in practice only those who had the necessary skills, abilities and experience regularly undertook.

Pelling's multi-dimensional view of sick-nursing means that she incorporates a large number of contemporary work-related and attendance-related terms and descriptions. As she points out, the word 'nurse' itself only became applicable to sick-nursing contexts in the seventeenth century. The terms 'keeping', 'tending' and 'looking-to' have to be considered as descriptions of attending the sick. These in turn lead the reader to a broad range of functions expressed in the provisions of the London hospitals: watching, providing food, cleaning clothes, cleaning rooms and houses, cleaning bodies (where necessary) and moral supervision. Such functions incurred negative connotations for the women who performed them: cleaning meant that nurses were associated with dirt as well as cleanliness, and attending those

6   Pelling, *Common lot*, 179–80.

with diseases inflamed the image of the nurse as a woman spreading infection. That sick nurses were normally strangers to urban patients (through
force of circumstance) exacerbated this image: nurses as 'uncaring' carers
compared to the more trustworthy 'caring' of wives and other close relatives. The very independence of nurses and their position of control *vis à vis*
the patient, Pelling argues, was a further destabilising threat and an added
reason for demeaning references in the contemporary literature. Low status,
or sufferance, was the (perhaps inevitable) consequence of such negative and
threatening connotations, giving rise to satire and obloquy. But through such
negatives Pelling shows that the sick-nurse existed as an occupation-related
identity (if not exactly an occupational one), in towns at least, at the beginning of the seventeenth century.

In 'Nurses and nurse-keepers' Pelling propounds an expansion of the definition of 'nursing' to include a wide range of functions. This raises some
interesting questions. One of the most important arguments which can be
advanced against an all-inclusive definition of medical practitioners – that
problems of identity mean that provision of medicines, and thus consumption of medicines, may be conflated with medical knowledge – may also be
brought against a view of sick-nursing which seeks to widen 'nursing' help to
all its constituent functions, for example washing and house-cleaning. Also,
just as some medical practitioners were less knowledgeable than others, or at
least less medically knowledgeable, so too some nurses would have been less
knowledgeable, and perhaps less medical, than others. However, it is worth
observing that, while an all-inclusive definition of medical assistance may
be justified through demonstrating a direct relationship between the practitioner and the ill person, an all-inclusive definition of sick-nursing is much
harder to justify in instances where the nurse or attendant was also attending
to the surroundings of the sick, and may not have been concerned with the
ill person at all. This is best exemplified by payments in the probate accounts
for cleaning which are impossible to classify as sick-nursing, especially when
the accounts include many payments for cleaning after the death. They may
have related to domestic chores requiring skill and expertise – drudgery is
not without its own set of skills and abilities – but they do not necessarily
relate to the tending of the sick.

Presumably because of such ambiguities, Pelling steered clear of attempting
a quantitative assessment of nursing availability along the lines of that undertaken in 1979 for medical practitioners. However, a numerical breakdown
of potential nurses is an important and necessary exercise, especially in the
light of rural services. There were about 290 parishes and substantial non-
parochial areas in East Kent, with a late seventeenth-century population
of between 76,000 and 95,000.[7] This gives an average parish population of

---

[7] A figure as high as 100,000 is not impossible: see chapter 2 above. The figure of 95,000
is derived from the Hearth Tax books of 1690.

260–325, of which roughly half would have been female. The average area covered by a parish was three square miles. To establish the number of skilled and experienced women in each square mile of East Kent, all the men and approximately 40 per cent of the females as under age must be discounted, leaving 78–97 adult women per parish, or 26–32 per square mile. It is true that this is probably an underestimate of the adult females available. A check is to divide the number of adults in the East Kent Compton Census returns (59,654) by the number of parishes represented therein (259), which gives an average parish population of over-sixteens of 230, i.e. 115 adult females.[8] If just 10 per cent of these women was aged 16–20, then on average there were 104 women over twenty-one, per parish. Not all of these women were free to attend the sick. With birth rates of roughly thirty per thousand, one in ten adult women would have had a child in the last year, and probably at least thirty per cent would have at least one child under the age of five. Assuming that women with young children had domestic priorities which precluded them serving their fellow parishioners, especially for sustained periods, the available adult female labour force numbered 54–73 women per parish, or 18–24 per square mile, and several of these – perhaps between three and five per square mile – would have been very aged or infirm.[9] Finally it should be noted that these figures have all included urban areas of high-density population along with the low-density rural areas. Therefore the rural levels of available female help were even lower. Bearing all this in mind, the number of near-neighbours upon whom one could call for potentially protracted periods of nursing help in rural areas was not large, probably no more than fifty within a mile of the average house. Finally, these figures do not take into consideration any of the other priorities women may have had, such as agricultural or other work, caring for ill people within their own homes, washing within the home and further afield, provision of food at home and further afield, and suchlike.

The reason for determining these figures is that a model of labour based on skills and experience must also take into consideration unskilled labour. Whatever skills are being considered, if there is no 'unskilled' labour in a parish, then the least-skilled person is comparatively 'unskilled'. Since every able-bodied sane person may be said to have had skills of one sort or another, the skills themselves were merely relative, and the very concept of sections of the population as 'skilled' may be seen to have been socially constructed. In this light, the whole labour pool may be seen to have consisted of people with a range of skills, many of whom in theory could have acted as nurses. So an approximate number of experienced able-bodied women available to act as nurses in that labour pool may be established. In the average East Kent

---

[8] In several East Kent parishes this figure also includes under-sixteens, and hence may be taken as an over-estimate.
[9] P. Laslett, *The world we have lost further explored*, London 2000, 111, gives 9% of the population in the seventeenth century as over sixty.

parish with fewer than twenty active women over the age of twenty-one per square mile, there would have been as many as thirty-five able-bodied males over the age of sixteen, a number of girls between sixteen and twenty-one, and a number of children. Thus those females who were ideal 'nurses' constituted a minority of the potential local labour force. Those who were prepared to do so (given the negative connotations of acting as a nurse, the dangers of infection, other demands on their time and labour, and the opprobrium in which some nurses were held) it would have been an even smaller minority.[10] In rural areas this very strongly supports Pelling's key point: that, if middle-aged women were attending as nurses, they were not drawn from some huge mass of unskilled and otherwise unemployed women, but rather the opposite: they were representative of a relatively small – and thus special – part of the labour force.

Before turning from 'Nurses and nurse-keepers' one other observation may be made. Its most important findings are not the consistencies of nurses and nursing but the inconsistencies, and the ambiguities. Just as chapter 4 stressed that a man who was qualified as a surgeon could be described by his various clients as a doctor, bloodletter, physician or even an apothecary, and that such inconsistencies of description were the norm, not the exception, so too the multiple and inconsistent descriptions of those who acted as nurses were normal. A woman might 'nurse', or she might 'wash', 'keep', 'watch' or 'look to' as well as a series of other less frequently found descriptions, and for her to be described as performing any or all of these functions was normal. In line with this definition-defying range of nursing activities, Pelling observes that men also undertook some nursing-related activities, and that in 'some "acute" situations involving infectious disease' a wide range of expedients could be employed, including taking back old servants as helpers, or using servants to administer first aid, or bringing washerwomen into a household. These ambiguities and inconsistencies may be approached in a number of ways. While it is entirely appropriate in 'Nurses and nurse-keepers' that they demonstrate how 'nursing' (broadly defined) was composed of irregular elements, in this study they must also be fitted into a definition of nursing care which permits quantification and comparison. Thus they raise a series of questions. To what extent did status affect who served as a nurse? Did servants regularly attend the dying? To what extent was nursing a female-dominated activity?

Pelling's multi-dimensional approach does not lend itself to a definition which can be applied systematically to the probate accounts. In fact to try to define 'sick-nursing' in the early modern period is something of an anachronism. It is true that the word 'nurse' was used, and that in certain contexts, especially after 1620, it might mean much the same as it does today, but, as

---

[10] For criticism of nurses harbouring plague cases see P. Slack, *Impact of plague in Tudor and Stuart England*, London 1985, 40.

Pelling's work shows, it can only be fully examined in an early modern sense by conflating a number of services and descriptions, and by paying specific attention to terms such as 'keep', 'tend' and 'watch', which do not necessarily relate to sick-nursing. The problems of definition are amplified by the overlaps which existed between nursing and medical care. A medical practitioner might be recorded as working in a nursing capacity, especially if he was 'watching' a patient following an operation. [11] Conversely, women who 'nursed' might have acted in a medical capacity, as in the case of the female medical practitioners referred to at the end of chapter 4. Thus, it has to be accepted that if nursing and medical assistance are to be separated, then a line of definition has to be drawn between them, and it is not possible to do this without prejudice to one or both sides. One shades into the other, like the blue of a rainbow shading into the red, and, to take the rainbow analogy a step further, it would necessitate discussing purple twice: once in the context of red and once in the context of blue. As a result any discussion of nursing which incorporates a discussion of medicine must draw some lines of demarcation. In this study, everything which could safely be regarded as matching the definition of 'medical' has been treated in the previous chapters. The result is that, in investigating 'nursing', it is the purchase of caring (broadly defined) that is being analysed; the element which may be defined by practitioner occupation, the administration of physic and attempted cures, has been removed. This approach is not favoured by most writers on the subject of nursing, who prefer to discuss 'nursing' and female medical care together from the slightly narrower point of view of women's roles within and outside the home, a perspective which allows nursing and healing easily to be conflated within the realm of women's work. However, the approach favoured here – separating the medical and the palliative – does have some significant advantages in that it makes it possible to quantify and contextualise the paid nursing undertaken by men, and avoids the pitfall of conflating the remedial and the palliative aspects of paid female assistance to the seriously ill and dying as if both these might be undertaken by nurses with equal readiness.

This approach depends primarily on the contemporary language used in the accounts. Nursing may be defined as caring services rendered to the dying which do not equate with the provision of 'medicines' or 'physic', which were not provided by an occupationally defined medical practitioner and which do not relate to an overt attempt to heal a specific malady. That said, certain exceptions need to be emphasised. First, while cleaning has been examined when it appears in conjunction with the purchase of other nursing services (for example 'paid for watching and cleaning in the time of the sickness'), isolated references to the cleaning of clothes or bedding

---

[11] Pelling, *Common lot*, 199–200. See also the reference to a surgeon 'watching' with the deceased, given later in the text.

have not been taken to be indicative of assistance to the dying. Second, it must be stressed that, by defining 'medical' purely in terms of occupational designation, remedial objective and medical substances, the possible medical aspects of services performed by those who were described as 'tenders' and 'attendants', who may have been so described in this way purely on account of their gender are inevitably neglected. In other words, it must be remembered that, if a physician administered a common herb to a dying man and the account described the act as 'Paid to the physician for physic administered', the act would be regarded as a medical one, whereas if an 'attendant' did this, and if it was described as 'help' or 'necessaries', not 'physic', that act would be regarded as a nursing one. The difference lies in the words used and the occupational designation of the practitioner, not the act itself. But to second-guess what services may or may not have led to an account entry and to make judgements on their medical content with no further evidence is not justifiable.

Quantifying household and family help

The overwhelming bulk of nursing care was provided freely by close members of the patient's family or household and thus, being free, does not appear in the accounts. It is important also to stress that the paid/unpaid differential did not necessarily equate with quality of care; a line cannot be drawn between unpaid and paid attendance and the latter regarded as somehow more expert than the former, or vice versa.[12] So although the probate sources almost completely ignore unpaid and domestic assistance, we may not. Rather the first step is to attempt to assess the level of nursing care which is not reflected in the accounts. Having done this, we may then examine what the accounts reveal about the nature of paid nursing care on behalf of the dying, returning at the end of the chapter to consider the implications for the unstated home and household help which is here quantified.

Since the majority of those paid to help the dying were women, by examining male patients an attempt may be made to catch a glimpse of the women in the household who may have attended the dying without charge. There are 11,617 accounts for men in the period 1570–1720 (excluding the 1650s). In 7,654 cases the accountant was female. In 6,748 of these cases the relationship of the female in question to the deceased is known: twenty-two creditors of the deceased, two aunts, one cousin, 209 daughters, five daughters-in-law, two granddaughters, thirteen female guardians of the deceased's children (often a sister or aunt), eighty-four mothers, four nieces, 183 sisters, three sisters-in-law, one stepmother and 6,219 widows. Excluding

---

12 Paul Slack's work on self-help books, indicating a readership in excess of 100,000, may point to some home-help being medically better informed than paid nursing care: 'Mirrors of health and treasures of poor men: the use of the vernacular medical literature of Tudor England', in Webster, *Health, medicine and mortality*, 9–60.

Table 56
Nursing and attendance services in relation to sex of administrators in East Kent

	A or B males with female executors/ administrators %	A or B males with male executors/ administrators %	C or D males with female executors/ administrators %	C or D males with male executors/ administrators %
1570–1649	11	20	9	22
1660–1720	13	21	12	21

the twenty-two creditors, in practically all cases the accountant – normally the next of kin – was a close relative of the patient, and in 92 per cent of cases was the man's wife. If the levels of nursing purchases in these cases is compared with those in which the executor or administrator was male, it is possible to estimate how regularly households with a female next of kin (who probably undertook some degree of attendance herself) made do without external care.

In the period 1570–1649, males with female next of kin paid for nursing care only half as regularly as those whose next of kin was male. It is probable that the households of married men were different from those of unmarried men with regard to staff, family and other dependants,[13] but all other things being equal, it is reasonable to assume that the discrepancy between these figures is directly attributable to the next-of-kin being female: that is to say, to her own attendance and that of any of her servants and companions who would not normally be found in the household of a man without a female next of kin. Thus with respect to higher status males in the period 1570–1649, it might be estimated that (100 per cent – 55 per cent) = 45 per cent of the attendance which would otherwise have been performed by paid helpers from outside the household was undertaken by the female next of kin or her servants. With respect to lower status males in the same period (100 per cent – 43 per cent) = 57 per cent of nursing attendance may be attributed to the presence of the female next of kin. These proportions seem to have declined slightly in the later period, to 38 per cent (higher status men) and 41 per cent (lower status men) as more external assistants were brought in to help with last illnesses.

The exactness of the above figures might give the impression that they are accurate assessments of care within the household. They are not. For example, these figures only relate to cases in which paid nursing help was completely absent, and thus to instances of the female next of kin presumably taking on all – not just most or some of – the attendance, albeit in some instances in

13 Mortimer, 'Medical assistance', i. 108–11.

conjunction with family, servants and unpaid helpers. Hence they must be considered absolute minima for estimates of wifely nursing. What, nevertheless, are the implications of these estimates? First, a figure of about 6 per cent should be allowed in respect of those men who died suddenly and who could not have benefited from nursing care to any significant degree.[14] Of higher status men who left a widow in the period 1570–1649, it is known that at least 11 per cent purchased nursing care, which, together with the 6 per cent of 'drop-dead' cases, leaves a maximum of 83 per cent who were exclusively attended by their family and household staff alone. From the above figures it would appear that more than half of this attendance (>45 per cent/<83 per cent = >54 per cent) was attributable to the presence of a female next of kin, with the rest of the household providing the remainder. In reality the boundaries would not have been so hard and fast: household staff probably attended in every case (if only along the lines of a household work model), and probably assisted paid helpers and the sick man's wife when they took part in the nursing process. The important point is that, even in a higher status household, the level of attendance attributable to the presence of a female next of kin, normally a wife, is very much greater than the recorded levels of paid outside attendance in these accounts. Although the wealthy could afford to hire many more helpers to assist with the dying patient, they also were able to rely on a larger body of household helpers, and so did not necessarily need to employ external help. But in all this the role of the wife, or other female kin, remained of prime importance.

For married men in the lower status groups this was even more noticeable. If 6 per cent of men died suddenly, and at least 9 per cent of patients received paid nursing care, then up to 85 per cent of care was provided exclusively by the household and family itself. Based on minimum estimates of female next-of-kin involvement, it is probable that in more than two-thirds of cases this is attributable to the presence of the sick man's wife (>57 per cent/<85 per cent = >67 per cent). These figures demonstrate that, although paid nursing is certainly under-recorded in these accounts, it could not have equalled the level of care expended on the dying man by his wife, family, servants and friends who gave their services freely. Since the bulk of the population in the period 1570–1649 would have fallen into what here have been classed status

---

[14] It is possible roughly to estimate the proportion of sudden deaths by comparing the proportions of testators' and intestates' accounts which do not mention nursing or medicine (both as broadly defined as possible) in the time of sickness: 76% of intestate males' accounts do not mention paid medical or nursing assistance compared to 65% of testators' accounts. Thus the proportion of men who died before they were sufficiently aware of their fate to make a written will was probably about 11%. The same calculation on accounts with nuncupative wills reveals a level halfway between this (as one would expect), with 70% showing no sign of medical and nursing help. Taking the difference between the intestate and the nuncupative levels, it might be estimated that roughly 6% of the sample of male patients died too soon to make a nuncupative will, and 5% died slowly enough to make a nuncupative will but too quickly to make a written one.

groups C and D (with chattels worth less than £100), should sick-nursing be understood as a major form of paid female employment or (as seems more likely) was it largely an unpaid female social obligation?

The language of nursing

Turning to an examination of payments, the language used in respect of all types of paid help may be considered. The logical starting point is the word 'nurse'. Both as a verb and a noun, this originally referred to the nursing of children. It seems often to have been understood in the context of 'nourishing' children in the late sixteenth and early seventeenth centuries, as some spellings suggest ('Paide for the Nourshing of the saide childe' being one example).[15] Some early references to nursing which appear to indicate sick-nursing have been identified,[16] but in the main the term 'nursing' is generally understood to relate to the wet- or dry-nursing of children until the seventeenth century.

This statement of changing meaning is, of course, a generalisation which takes no note of regional variation. In East Kent it is possible to be more systematic since there are at least five hundred references specifically to 'nurses' or 'nursing' between 1578 and 1726, and where these relate to the nursing of children it is usually possible to differentiate between them and sick-nursing, due to the necessity of justifying payments on behalf of beneficiaries in probate accounts. The only sixteenth-century reference in which 'nursing' appears in any context which might relate to sickness is a 1599 reference to nursing Rebecca Buckhurst, who was a child.[17] The first entry which might relate to nursing a man in his sickness is dated 1601 and mentions that a female 'nurse' was paid for 'attending' the deceased and his widow and children.[18] The next entry relating to nursing as a sickness activity, dated 1608, also has connotations of child-nursing, as the reference to the nurse appears alongside a reference to a midwife attending on John Clay and his wife.[19] There are further references to 'nursing' in a context of adult sickness coupled with child care in the early seventeenth century, in which the latter might have influenced the language used, and several appearances of the term 'nurse' as a pretitle ('Nurse Alcocke') or epithet ('a certain poore woman, a nurse'). The earliest reference to a 'nurse' devoid of

---

[15] All the specific 'nursing' references found in East Kent accounts for 1578–1726 are transcribed in Mortimer, 'Medical assistance', ii. 122–42.

[16] Pelling, *Common lot*, 185–6. Note that the two early references therein to Mr Malory and Mr Daniells are not necessarily references to adults in the contexts quoted, as the 'Mr' could be an indicator of status as opposed to maturity.

[17] PRC 2/10/450.

[18] PRC 2/12/66.

[19] PRC 2/14/110.

connotations of infant dependency is dated 1609: 'paide vnto Nurse Ivers of the towne of Sandwich for watching and attending with and vppon the saide testator John Crispe in the time of the sickness whereof he died'.[20] Nursing references relating to adult sickness are to be found in the 1620s but are not common until after 1660.

Given the shift in the language used in East Kent, it is necessary to identify what alternatives were used to describe nursing functions at earlier dates, and the regularity with which these terms were used. This is not as easy as it seems, partly because the original indexing did not necessarily associate cleaning, 'helping' or 'keeping' in the time of sickness with illness or medicine (the two indexing terms used), and partly because some of the terms themselves are interwoven with other language and subtexts. In some cases there are references to attendance by physicians separate from attendance by nurses, but in others there are composite payments for 'physic and attendance' without indication as to whether the attendance relates to the presence of a medical practitioner supplying physic or someone supplying nursing care (and possibly also obtaining physic). Nevertheless, it is possible to derive approximate comparative figures to illustrate the regularity of the descriptions of services.

Tables 57 and 58 suggest a number of changing features of the word 'nursing'. The first and most obvious is that references to 'nursing/nurses' are predominantly found in post-Restoration documents. More than half of all references to 'attendance', 'tending' and 'looking after/to' after 1660 are to be associated with 'nurses' and 'nursing', compared to less than 2 per cent before the Interregnum. It is also clear that, while assistance in preparing the corpse for burial was often coupled with the service of attending or watching, this was less common when the assistant was described as a 'nurse' or paid for 'nursing'. Other features include the disappearance of the use of the word 'keeping' after the Restoration, and the steady decline throughout the period in the use of the word 'watching', two service descriptions which are most strongly associated with helpers who were not described as 'nurses'.

The changes so described were not related to patients' status. Indeed, the nomenclature of nursing shows a remarkable consistency across all the status groups (see table 59). Every status group in the period 1570–1609 was slightly more likely to describe nursing assistance in terms of 'watching' than 'attendance'. In every status group this was reversed in the following period, as 'watching' declined as a description. After the Restoration, 'watching' became obsolete, or rendered of negligible importance as a description, and 'attendance' also significantly declined. 'Keeping' declined to zero in every group. And finally, in every status group, 'nursing' as a service descriptor (or 'nurse', as a description of an attendant) became more important in the post-1660 period. The language may thus be seen to have had the same currency

<hr />

[20] PRC 2/15/66.

Table 57
Regularity of descriptions of assistance in conjunction with 'nurse' or 'nursing'

Services specified	1570–1609	1610–49	1660–99
'Attendance', 'tending' and 'looking after/to' and 'nursing'	4?	12	355
'Helping'	0	0	0
'Keeping'	1	1	0
'Watching'	2	1	19
Wetnursing/drynursing	28	13	9
Cleaning [in conjunction with the above]	0	0	6
Funeral assistance [in conjunction with the above]	0	1	27

Table 58
Regularity of descriptions of nursing services used in conjunction with individuals not described as 'nurses' or paid for 'nursing'

Services specified	1570–1609	1610–49	1660–99
'Attendance', 'tending' and 'looking after/to'	338	784	210
'Helping'	10	18	9
'Keeping'	69	36	0
'Watching'	383	419	62
Wetnursing/drynursing	28	13	9
Cleaning [in conjunction with the above]	54	70	17
Funeral assistance [in conjunction with the above]	50	158	45

across the board, among all types of accountants, from the rich to the poor, when filtered through the process of the court clerk making the official copy.

The rise and fall in the use of certain words across time periods begs the important question of whether the actual activities undertaken by assistants were changing, or just the means of describing them (for example, the language of the court clerk). Were 'nurses' more medicalised than 'helpers'? Or was the word simply reflecting a more coherent concept of the role of the bedside assistant? Did people stop 'watching' in about 1700–20, or were the watchers then described as 'nurses'? Were 'keepers' after 1660 described as nurses? These questions are similar to those already faced in respect of providers of physic and surgeons; but, ironically, are easier to handle because of the very lack of practitioner identities in nursing assistance. Whereas descriptions of medical payments often refer to practitioners' occupational

Table 59
Proportions of nursing designations in respect of each status group

Specified services	Status A and equivalent Status R) %	Status B (and equivalent Status R) %	Status C (and equivalent Status S) %	Status D (and equivalent Status S) %
'Attendance', 'tending' and 'looking after/to' performed by non-'nurses'				
1570–1609	14	11	9	9
1610–49	13	11	16	12
1660–99	5	5	6	7
'Attendance', 'tending', 'looking after/to' performed by 'nurses', including 'nursing'				
1660–99	10	10	9	10
'Watching' by non-'nurses'				
1570–1609	16	13	12	9
1610 49	6	7	7	7
1660–99	2	2	2	1
'Keeping' performed by non-'nurses'				
1570–1609	2	3	1	2
1610–49	0.1	1	0.5	1

identity rather than medical activity (for example 'paid the surgeon'), the relative paucity of nursing identities means that a description of activities is more frequently included. In other words, those paid for nursing services were described more often by their services than by a medical identity.

'Attendance', 'tending' and 'looking after/to'

The terminology of attendance (excluding 'keeping', 'watching' and 'helping') is dominated by two types of words: those involving 'tending/attending' and those involving 'looking'. These types are not mutually exclusive: entries such as 'paid to a poore woman for looking to & attendinge vppon the saide Clarckes wife in the tyme of the sicknes whereof she dyed' are by no means

147

uncommon.[21] Throughout the period the dominant term is 'tending'. Laying aside all references which incorporate mention of nurses or nursing, and those entries which are exclusively for helping, keeping or watching, 91 per cent of the attendance references in the period 1570–1649 include nouns or verbs with the root 'tend'. In the period 1660–99, 80 per cent of payments were for services based on 'tend'. In the early eighteenth century 'tending' diminished in frequency, and 'looking' increased, to 50 per cent and 33 per cent respectively.

In total there are 1,332 non-nursing payments which may be included in a survey of 'attendance' (including 'looking to/after'), 1,122 of which fall before 1650. Only six are to people with a designation of higher social status, described as 'Mrs'.[22] By comparison, fifty-two payments were made to people described as 'poor', all of which pre-date the Interregnum, and 122 were made to women described as widows (eighty-seven of which pre-date 1650). Women described as 'Goodwife [+ surname]' or 'Goody [+ surname]' account for a further 107 payments, and women described as being their husband's wife another 105. While many of the remainder may have been poor and/or wives/widows as well, the evidence regarding identities suggests that paid non-nursing attendance was provided by various marital groups (maids, married men and women, and widows, and possibly single men) and a range of people from the poor to the perceived-to-be-solvent, from old widows to married women, but not often the wealthy, the gentle or those marked by designations of elevated social respectability.

The sense of communities supplying people to tend the seriously ill and dying is strengthened by an examination of the geographical backgrounds of the tenders. There are 113 assistants not described as 'nurses' or paid for 'nursing' whose home parishes are given in these accounts. Table 60 indicates how regularly the dying sought help from people of their own parishes.

Since the figures include cases of people who died away from home – two died in London – they may be considered good evidence that fellow parishioners were of considerable importance in providing attendance. In many cases where the assistant was from another parish, it was normally adjacent

---

[21] PRC 2/7/117. Nor are these terms exclusive with regard to keeping, helping or watching.

[22] These six are (1) 'paid to Mrs Swift for lookinge to the saide deceased in the time of his sickness': PRC 2/21/55, dated 1620; (2) 'to Mrs Lewkner wyef of Alexander Lewkner for her paynes she tooke with him in the time of his sicknes, and which hee willed to bee giuen unto her towardes the buyinge of a Cowe': PRC 20/6/312, dated 1623; (3) 'to Mrs Jarvis for attending the said deceased in the time of his sicknes': PRC 20/8/33, dated 1628; (4) 'paid vnto Mrs Nightingale for her attendance on the said deceased in his sicknes': PRC 2/37/162, dated 1677; (5) 'paid more to the said Mrs Oxenden for board and dyett for the said deceased with his watchers and other attendants from the 27th of September 1678 to 14th of February next following being in his time of sicknes and weakened': PRC 2/39/127, dated 1680; (6) 'paid to Mrs Wilson for looking after the deceaseds widow in the time of the sickness': PRC 19/5/66, dated 1700.

Table 60
Location of non-nursing assistants attending
and helping the dying in East Kent

Date	Proportion from same parish as deceased (urban parishes, <1m)	Proportion from same parish as deceased (rural parishes)	All parishes
1570–1609	1/1	19/26	20/27 (74%)
1610–49	22/25	40/54	62/79 (78%)
1660–1720	3/4	2/3	5/7 (71%)

to that of the deceased.[23] When it is noted that the accounts were biased towards recording the homeplaces of more distant practitioners (in order to justify greater costs), the importance of the parish community becomes even more pronounced. Other social details support this still further. Members of the Dutch congregations in Sandwich and Canterbury attended each other (for example, Lothe Maes attended Charles Vanhuele, and John Wermentin attended Francis Casteker).[24] But despite this, parish communities should not be confused with personal connections, nor taken as an indication that the people attending in these cases were friends of, or even known to, the deceased. Contemporary – usually town-dwelling – playwrights stressed the strangeness of the women who nursed them,[25] but rural administrators too were often unaware of the names of – and presumably unfamiliar with – the people who attended their dead kin. Through systematically recording the names left blank in these accounts it can be shown that in at least thirty-two cases the accountant did not know part of the name of the attendant at

[23] Examples being 'paide to Glovers widow of Smarden for looking vnto and tending vppon the saide Joan Finckle [of Headcorn] in the tyme of her sicknes', 1594: PRC 2/7/59; and 'paid to Sara Skivington of Lyd for her watching with the deceased [of Old Romney] in the tyme of her sicknes whereof she dyed', 1601: PRC 2/13/254; and 'paide to one woordes wife of Stodmershe for her paynes in attending on the saide testatorix [of Wickhambreaux] in the tyme wherof shee dyed', 1604: PRC 2/12/78. Other, more distant assistants are represented by entries such as 'paide to goodwife Tucker of Canterburye for attending on the testatorix [of Wickhambreaux] all the tyme of the sicknes wherof shee dyed', 1604: PRC 2/13/42; and 'paide by this Accomptante vnto a poore woman of ffeversham for weching [watching] with the said John Wheeler deceassed [of Eastchurch Sheppey] in the time of his sickness.', 1605: PRC 2/14/494; and 'paid to the wydowe Peers of the saide parishe of mylton for chardges and expences made and due by the said intestate [of Blean] in the time of his sickness ..., lyinge sicke a fortnight and more or thereabowtes beefore his deathe', 1609: PRC 2/14/329.
[24] PRC 2/17/426, PRC 2/17/434. Ann Hess observed that non-Quaker 'parish midwives' and other non-Quaker women attended Quaker births. She noted that non-Quaker involvement ran at about 32%. However, there was very probably a shortage of Quaker midwives in rural communities, which would explain the difference: 'Midwifery practice among the Quakers', 53.
[25] See Pelling, Common lot, 201.

the time of rendering the account, even though the attendant was a fellow parishioner. 'Paid to Dennis [blank] of Mersham for the like her paynes taken' is one example of part of the name of an attendant from the same parish being unknown to the accountant;[26] 'paid to [blank] Johnson of Birchington for attending upon the deceased Thomas Clarke in the tyme of the sicknes' is another.[27] The same might be said of some payments which do not leave blanks, such as: 'paid to one Simpsons widow for watching'.[28] In very many more no name is given at all, 'certain women' being a very common descriptor, probably covering many other cases where the attendants were not known to the accountant. Since most of the instances of partially-recalled names pre-date the Interregnum it would appear that, before 1650 at least, it was the wider parish community which undertook attendance activities, not just local friends and relatives of the deceased.

If the wider community could be called upon to assist in the care of the dying, to what extent did this involve men? This is a contentious subject, on account of attempts by some writers to emphasise the importance of women's medical assistance before the rise of hospital-trained medical practitioners. This in itself – although heavily based on presumptions about unpaid care – is not unreasonable, given the importance of medical knowledge in the home, but it is unreasonable to assume that attendance at the bedside was exclusively carried out by women, as writers stressing the 'feminized locale' of the deathbed have done.[29] While there is no doubt that sick-nursing was generally considered more appropriate for women than men as an occupation, it is equally clear that men did take a share in the bedside attendance of the dying.[30] Indeed it might be argued that in extraordinary circumstances men could be expected to provide extraordinary support as readily (if not as often) as women, well beyond their usual gender-typified roles.

Payments for male assistance – while much less common than payments to women – are not hard to find. There are about 130 payments to males for keeping, watching, looking to/after, attending and helping in times of sickness (about 6 per cent of all recorded instances of these words). However, there are significant differences between male and female attendance. Obviously, it was a little unusual to employ a male attendant, as the low figure of 6 per cent shows. Men usually only attended other men whereas women tended both sexes. Possibly this was because of the suspicion of impropriety

26 PRC 2/12/308.
27 PRC 20/1/268.
28 PRC 2/6/201. It must be borne in mind that such 'distant' references might possibly reflect a conscious distancing on account of social or status differences.
29 Mendelson and Crawford, *Women in early modern England*, 210.
30 With regard to the appropriateness of women in a nursing role see PRC 2/32/5, dated 1633. This is worded 'for attendance and women's helpe in the deceasedes last sicknes', thereby stressing the female nature of the help, not just the fact that it was work which happened to be performed by women. Another example is PRC 2/32/109, which reads 'for women's attendance and helpe in the said deceaseds sicknes and at his funerall'.

on the part of a man in a position of power over an ill (and perhaps defence-less) woman, but also it may be because of the limitations on the kin and friendship networks of some administrators (as discussed later in relation to 'watching'). In some cases men and women tended a female patient together, as with 'William Owlett and [blank] his wife of Boughton Munchelsey aforesaid for their paines and labour on tending and watching with the said deceased in the time of the sickness whereof she died'.[31] But male/female couplings were not always husband and wife teams: John Crayford and Widow Matthewes were paid in 1637 'for watching with and attendance on the said deceased Agnes, John and Thomas Plott in the tymes of their said last sicknes'.[32] Where women were being tended, the male tender was nearly always accompanied by a female.[33]

A third difference between male and female attendance was that of phys-ical strength. Some people did not die 'a good death' but, in the words of Dylan Thomas, 'raged against the dying of the light'. One reference is poignantly clear on the subject: 'to one barber a man for attending the said deceased in his last contagious disease and helping to keep him in his bed and hold him he being very distressed some part of the time'.[34] Seclusion in one's home was not something to which everyone with a contagious illness acqui-esced. Nor did the problem just arise from men trying to escape their houses, as one 1639 account from Brenzett shows.[35] Where men were employed in respect of attending mental derangement or delirium, their presence might be merely protection for a female helper, as possibly reflected in the 1674 entry, '[paid] to a man and a woman for attending a week night and day in the time of his said last sickness he being all that time much troubled and distracted in his mind'.[36] In other cases, especially smallpox, the disease was the stated justification for male attendants being employed, possibly implying the reluctance of the deceased to remain confined in his own house in that particular case but also possibly implying a regular male attendance function, as in 'paid unto the men tendors of the said deceased hee dying of the small pox' (Charing, 1641).[37] In support of this (and contrary to usual understand-ings of the disease), it may be said that non-occupational male attendance

[31] PRC 2/21/125, dated 1617: the attendants were from the same parish as the sick woman.

[32] PRC 20/11/242.

[33] But note the entry in PRC 2/9/281: 'paide vnto Richard Patching of Rolvinden for chardges due to him for attendance on the saide deceassed in the tyme of her sicknes and other expences therabowte'. Perhaps some women were felt to be safe from single, unaccompanied male attendance, possibly due to a number of servants in the house, or family relations.

[34] PRC 1/8/59, dated 1649.

[35] PRC 1/3/49. The entry reads 'paid to two men for their continual attendance on him in the time of his last sickness for a fortnight with their diet he being frantic'.

[36] PRC 1/1/48.

[37] PRC 19/2/28.

on smallpox victims is regularly found in these accounts.[38] Furthermore, most male 'tending' entries are worded in such a way that it is reasonably clear that the men were not being employed as watchmen, with a responsibility to make sure the deceased did not escape, although their presence within the house may well have served much the same function. A few are ambiguous,[39] but those payments which were to watchmen are normally very clear, for example 'paid unto Thomas Robinson who was imployed as a watchman to attend upon the said visited by the space of 14 weeks for his wages after the rate of seven shillings per week'.[40] Leaving aside all payments to watchmen, about a third of all male attendance cases are in some way attributable to a special aspect of the illness, whether it be violence, mental derangement or smallpox. The remainder include no justification for male employment and thus imply that no justification was felt to be necessary. Men may have been employed in some cases in order that the tenders could move a particularly heavy patient in his sickness. It may reasonably be concluded that, before 1650 especially, male attendance was deemed essential in some circum-stances, and in many cases desirable, but normally those who were paid for tending the sick as attendants were women.[41]

If the majority of those attending the dying were females drawn from the local community, what factors conditioned their selection, especially when they were not known to the deceased and his family? Various text-book writers have proposed – and common sense supports – the existence of groups of experienced women who would move in and assist in the running of the household during a serious illness; and the practice of poor towns-

---

[38] In addition to the 1641 and 1649 examples given in this paragraph the following might be considered: 'payde to Alexander Stonestreete of Goodherst for looking to and attending on the saide deceassed ... hee beeing sicke of the infectious disease of the poxe': PRC 2/19/87, dated 1615; 'paid to one William Deframe for attending the deceased ... hee lying long visited with the small pockes of which visitation hee died': PRC 2/29/82, dated 1629; 'to two men which attended the said deceased in his sickness ... hee dying of the smallpoxe': PRC 2/33/36, dated 1635; 'to 4 men for attending the said deceased in the time of the sickness whereof hee dyed beeing of the small poxe And for their dyet and the dyett of a little girl for a monthes time after his death till they were thought to bee free from that disease': PRC 2/34/101, dated 1637; 'paid unto several men which attended upon the said deceased in his sickness ... he dying of a disease commonly called the smallpox': PRC 1/14/22, dated 1669; 'paid to William Goodsole for attending the deceased in his sicknes which was the small pox and the deceased so much distempered therewith that a woman could not rule him and for laying him forth in all': PRC 2/42/127, dated 1698; 'paid to John Moore for nurses and looking after the said deceased and his family in the time of his sickness whereof he died they being sick of the smallpox': PRC 1/17/43, dated 1711. For Margaret Pelling's suggestion that, far from being a male activity, female nursing of smallpox victims (often children) gave rise to the use of the word 'nurse' in sick-nursing contexts over the seventeenth century see *Common lot*, 198–9.

[39] See PRC 1/14/22 in n. 38 above;

[40] PRC 1/13/73.

[41] Of references to men in nursing roles (broadly defined) 121/140 (86%) predate 1650. By comparison 70% of all accounts in this study predate 1650.

women being called in to tend and generally assist poor urban families is well known.[42] But the real issue is whether the local women who performed the bulk of the attendance had some particular experience, skill or identity which resulted in their being selected for the task. Any ability to answer this question on the strength of the probate accounts evidence is hampered by the lack of any explicit references to medical or nursing skill or knowledge, but some observations are possible, and these are perhaps all the more valuable in that the identities and services of 'attendants' may thereby be compared with those of 'nurses'.

To begin with location, it is clear that attendants were sometimes drawn from neighbouring parishes. It is true that some attendants did travel a long way, but normally it is clear why they did so. Reasons are implicit in several entries, such as 'paid to Catherine Hemes for attending of the said Martha Vanhill deceased [of Sandwich] in the tyme of her sicknes whercof she dyed she dying of the plage & the charges of fetching of the said Catherine from Dover to that purpose',[43] and 'to the wydowe Joanes of Stourmouth for keeping the said deceaseds house [in Monkton] in order, for tending on the said deceased in the time of his said sicknes and yt being as aforesaid feared and suspected that the said deceased was infected with a Contagious disease'.[44] Where contagious illnesses were concerned, there may have been a reluctance to attend, especially as the attendant risked being incarcerated in the house for a month after the infection was cleared, assuming that she survived. There are only two instances in which attendants were sought from a greater distance than the adjacent parish for no apparent reason (excluding men dying in London and cases of wet-nursing). One of these was the payment 'to Widow Vane and Goodwife Downe of Lenham who helped at the house of the said intestate [in Hollingbourne] in his sicknes he dyed of'.[45] The other was the 1604 payment 'to goodwife Tucker of Canterburye for attending on the testatorix all the tyme of the sicknes wherof shee dyed'.[46] This Wickhambreaux patient also received attention from a woman from Stodmarsh, the next village, and so in sending to Canterbury for a female attendant as well, she falls more into the category of those employing women from medical towns for their specific medical skills (see chapter 4).

This militates against there having been a large mobile cadre of women with greater experience, skill or identity attending the dying outside the contexts of 'nursing'. However, it does not rule out the possibility of there being such a cadre within each parish. At this juncture it should be recalled

[42] With regard to the poor nursing the poor see Andrew Wear, 'Caring for the sick poor in St Bartholomew Exchange, 1580–1676', in R. Porter and W. Bynum (eds), Living and dying in London (Supplement to Medical History xi, 1991), 41–60.
[43] PRC 2/16/48.
[44] PRC 20/3/101.
[45] PRC 20/13/416.
[46] PRC 2/13/42.

that most attendants were women, and that the total proportion of able-bodied women aged 21–60 without children under the age of five was probably less than 20 per cent of the population, and the number of experienced women without other social and economic priorities who were able to take on attendance functions probably amounted to no more than half this. Thus, if there were experienced women within each parish who acted as nurses in cases of serious illness, they were drawn from a small group. In other words, when considering what factors conditioned the choice of nurse, there was probably in fact no 'choice' as such, but rather a shifting group of people who usually attended.

What of the monetary and related payments made to attendants? Fortunately, since accountants could not easily justify attendance payments in terms of occupational definition, they often resorted to quantifications of time. Nearly three hundred accounts include some indication of the length of time for which the deceased was sick or the period of attendance for which an individual was paid. By singling out those payments made for 'attendance' and 'looking after/to' (excluding those to 'nurses') the ranges of payments may be determined.[47] The usual payment for attendance in the period 1570–1609 appears to have been around 2s. per week per attendant, with two high payments (6s. 8d. and 8s. 2d. per week) at the start of the period, and lower payments of about 1s. per week in respect of the employment of poor women (9d. per week to one 'pore mayden'). Later accounts reveal set payments for attendance in respect of plague and smallpox at levels of 6s. 8d. and 8s. per week, and so it is likely that the two higher rates for the 1570s reflect unspecified contexts of contagious illness. In the period 1610–49 payments for attendance ranged from 1s. 6d. in respect of payments to 'poor women' to 10s. 6d., again an amount possibly predicated by an otherwise unmentioned contagious disease. Payments of 7s. (inclusive of diet) and 8s. per week were made in respect of two cases of continual attendance upon mentally ill patients.[48] At the other end of the spectrum, long-term attendance was comparatively cheap: the payment 'to certain women for attending the said deceased in the time of his sickness, he being sick the space of one whole year' merited a mere 45s.[49] In a very interesting account, dated 1636, a mother (Goodwife Dixon) and daughter were paid at almost the same rate for attending their fellow parishioner, Abdias Pownall: the mother was paid 2s. 5d. per week for three weeks; the daughter 2s. for six days.[50] This might indicate a girl gaining experience through working alongside her mother, but even if not, it shows a standard level of remuneration irrespective of age and experience. What emerges is a pattern of normal payments of about 2s. 6d.– 4s. per week for attendance (the higher rates possibly including

[47] Mortimer, 'Medical assistance', ii. 143–7.
[48] PRC 1/3/49, PRC 1/1/48.
[49] PRC 1/3/46. This could have been occasional attendance.
[50] PRC 2/34/99.

diet), but half of this (1s. 6d. per week) if the attendant were poor, and twice this (about 7s.–8s. per week) if the disease was contagious or otherwise threatening or unpleasant.

The pattern of payments suggests that a process of negotiation took place, starting from (and often ending at) the relevant amount in respect to the status of the attendant and the medical situation of the patient. This amount seems to have been adjusted on a case-by-case basis when the normal level was insufficient to attract an attendant, or when the period of attendance was expected to be extended. Clearly residential attendants also benefited from the food that they were given (the accounts give many totals of the food allowances for attendants, usually approximating to the equivalent of their wages and sometimes more), but it is equally clear that those in the weakest bargaining position had to accept the low wages set. This was the case even when the dying patient was rich: Widow Spencer's patient in 1693 had chattels worth £565, and still she was paid the standard 1s. 6d. per week (for thirteen weeks) for a poor woman, an amount which did not alter across the century. Thus the variation in amounts paid for attending may be attributable to three factors: (1) the status of attendants; (2) expectations of work required (largely based on the medical condition of the deceased); and (3) scarcity of nurses, in the light of the observations on the availability of female labour. The status of the deceased does not appear to have been a factor in determining levels of remuneration, in contrast to payments made for medical help.

The payment of higher wages in specific medical contexts raises another important question. Were these in respect of greater experience and skill, or discomfort in nursing the ill (as occurred at St Bartholomew's Hospital, where nurses on the disease or 'foul' wards were paid more) or were they because of the threat of the attendants themselves catching the illness?[51] There is no doubt that attendants did put themselves very much at risk, as the following 1605 reference reveals:

> Item these Accomptantes pray to be allowed the summe of 20s the which was paid to Margaret Dillnott a widow woman the which did attend upon the deceased William Chapman in the tyme of the sicknes whereof he died who was then also taken sicke & before such tyme as she could be recovered & the howse of the deceased discharged of the said Margaret the expenses made in the tyme of the same her sicknes did extend to the sum of 20s.[52]

Even more extraordinary is the case of Thomas Johnson, who acted as an attendant in a plague house prior to 1598, and caught the disease, so that his own house was boarded up. After his death his widow claimed for her

---

51 See V. Bullough and B. Bullough, *The care of the sick: the emergence of modern nursing*, London 1979, 58.
52 PRC 20/1/1. Other accounts which record that the attendant became infected include PRC 2/34/251 and PRC 2/16/172.

husband's 'paynes & hyndrance for the space of xiiii or xv weeks in attending one the parties aforesaid infected & supplying such things as they then wanted being thereby shunned of all men & hindred greatelie in his trade & worldlie dealings'.[53] But that was not all: the woman who tended him in his sickness also fell ill with plague, and required assistance. Such risks were presumably well-known to the attendant, and this was the reason for the higher weekly rates specified in the accounts. Rates at this level suggest pre-attendance agreements or contracts (almost certainly verbal), in the cases of plague and smallpox attendance at least.[54] These contracts may be said to presuppose that both the risks to and requirements of the attendants were known to both parties in advance of their agreement. If this were the case, then there is no reason on the evidence of the probate accounts to suppose that higher payments in respect of contagious illnesses were due to experience or risk factors but rather every reason to suspect they were agreed in respect of both experience and risk. This does not necessarily mean that there was a medical element to attendance on smallpox and plague cases which was reflected in the payments, but rather that, in contracting to attend a smallpox victim for a certain amount per week, a female attendant was bringing to the case an appreciation of the disagreeable and possibly life-threatening nature of the task, and that this was what differentiated her payment from a woman attending a man dying of 'old age'. This would explain why plague attendants sometimes travelled considerable distances.

One last feature of payments in respect of attendance is the practice of paying in kind. No particular circumstances seem to have governed such payments. Two 'poore women' were paid 'in money 18d and a wastcoate prized att 6d'.[55] The same account states that 'Bennetts wife of [blank]' was paid 'for helping to attende the saide deceased and his servants in the tyme of their severall sicknesses of the plague one cowe worth 40s'. Both of these entries suggest that the attendants were not part of the deceased's family circle. Friends might also be paid in kind, and a payment of a cow was even specified in a 1623 payment to one of the few women referred to as 'Mrs'.[56] Most payments in kind involved clothing, and not necessarily that in which the deceased died: 'to certaine woemen which did attend watch with and looke to the said deceased … in money xlvs and also so much of the apparell of the said deceased worth by comon estimacion the summe of

---

[53] PRC 2/10/340, dated 1598. This includes a payment for 'The bording & dyett of the said Catherine Johnson for vi weeks after she came out of the said howse infected.'

[54] These should not be taken to be 'contracts' in the sense that Margaret Pelling uses the term in Medical conflicts, but as more akin to informal agreements, such as those to perform seasonal agricultural work, for example.

[55] PRC 2/14/197.

[56] 'Mrs Lewkner wyef of Alexander Lewkner' was paid 'for her paynes she tooke with him in the time of his sicknes, and which hee willed to bee giuen unto her towardes the buyinge of a Cowe': PRC 20/6/206.

xls'.[57] Goodwife Goodridge was paid 'for her paynes in keeping and attending the said deceased in the tyme of her sicknes wherof she died a hatt prised at 2s 6d'.[58] In the pre-Commonwealth period especially, payment in kind seems to have been simply another form of remuneration which accountants made, in addition to promises of bequests made by the deceased themselves. There is no indication of attendants' rights over bedding or clothes after the death of the deceased beyond such payments; indeed several attendants were paid for washing the bedding and clothes of the dead, often as a prelude to it being sold.[59]

Drawing together these observations about paid non-nursing attendance, it may be said, with some confidence, that it seems to have been a local, largely female business, as most writers have assumed, and mostly performed by the less well-off. The exceptions lie in contagious illnesses and mental derangement, when local men and women from further afield were some-times employed on account of their strength, experience or acceptance of high risks. The key point is that, in the period when references to 'nursing' were rare, the people 'attending' and 'looking to/after' were very rarely sought from medical towns for their specific skills but were mostly local and paid at standard rates according to their own status and the requirements of the attendance in question (unless widespread diseases meant that they were otherwise engaged). If such attendance included a strong medical element, it was provided by local women who were employed for their availability (implying a lack of other priorities), their readiness in non-contagious cases to work for low wages (implying low-status skills which were not greatly valued or heavily in demand), their past experience (which, logically, must have mostly been gained locally) or a combination of all of these. None of these features is commensurate with a high level of remedial expertise or medical knowledge, even by contemporary standards, and it is a telling fact that only one female attendant is named in more than one account before 1650, suggesting that such women were not very regularly or exclusively employed even in their own parishes.[60] No woman was explicitly paid for

57 PRC 2/24/178.
58 PRC 2/11/294.
59 For example, 'paid vnto certeaine weomen that watched with the said deceased & his wife in the time of the sicknes wherof they dyed for socking [the Kentish word for shrouding] of them when they were dead and for washing such linnen & apparrell as was fowled in the time of their sicknes': PRC 2/17/105; and 'payd to such persons as did watch with and attend the testator Ambrose Cobb in the tyme of his sicknes wherof he dyed & did wasshe his linnen & did perform & do other necessarie thinges about his howse after his death': PRC 2/17/155, 153, 154. There are many such payments to attendants for washing the linen after the death.
60 This is Widow Alcock of Canterbury, who appears in two accounts dated 1610: 'Paid to wydow Alcocke one other of the keepers of the howse of the said deceased for her wages for ten weekes': PRC 2/15/277; and 'paide vnto nurse Alcocke, Goodwife Marple and Elizabeth Goldridge for their paines and attendance done to and on the saide dece-assedes famylie in the tyme of the visitacion': PRC 20/2/122.

her experience or skill in a non-nursing attendance context, and those who were paid for physic (*see* chapter 4) were very few in number. It is worth observing that many women paid for attendance seem to have been maid-servants paid for their household management experience, not their medical knowledge.[61] On this basis it may reasonably be concluded that there were parochial contingents of potential attendants in the late sixteenth and seventeenth centuries, mostly female, ranging from a small core of experienced able-bodied women (probably less than 10 per cent of the workforce, or an average of seven women per square mile) to a large number of household helpers with no remedial experience, the latter being employed along the lines of servant-maids and servants, to feed, clean and accompany the ill. The references to people employed in this way in the late sixteenth and early seventeenth centuries indicate that, unless they were attending contagious diseases, most attendants at this time were employed specifically for their domestic skills and additional labour (for example during the night-time), and were not required to have significantly greater medical knowledge than was commonly possessed by the average wife, widow or maidservant.

'Watching'

One specific service often described in conjunction with attendance was that of 'watching'. The word appears in more than 870 payments, almost all of which may be certainly associated with palliative care, although in rare cases the word appears with no medical or nursing context, and very occasionally payments to medical practitioners were recorded for watching.[62] As shown in tables 57 and 58, it was a term usually associated with non-nursing attendants, not with 'nurses' or 'nursing'. Furthermore, it was very much on the wane as 'nursing' descriptions increased. Prior to 1610 references to watching were as common as those to attending. In the four decades 1610–49 it was half as common, and after 1660 it was little more than a

---

[61] For example, 'to a woman and a maide which attended the said deceased': PRC 20/9/87, dated 1630; 'to the maid which attended the said deceased': PRC 2/29/26, dated 1628; 'paid to a woman & a maid for laying forth and watching with the deceased': PRC 2/32/121, dated 1634; 'paide to Susan Whitton a maide of the parish of Bonington afforesaid for [attending?] and watching with the said deceased': PRC 2/32/68, dated 1634: 'To John Brent for his maides iourney to fetch phisicke for the said Sybill and for watching with her in her aforesaid sicknes'; PRC 2/34/70, dated 1637; and 'paide to a maide servante of the howse wherein the saide testator laye sicke for attending on him in the tyme of his sicknes wherof hee dyed': PRC 2/13/356, dated 1603. There are many further references in these account to 'maids' and 'maid servants' being paid for attending and watching.

[62] A rare example of a medical practitioner 'watching' with the deceased is in the 1622 account of Alexander Norwood: 'payde to William Jorden a Chirurgion for letting the sayde deceased bloud and for watching with him that night': PRC 2/24/28.

quarter. There are only five references to watching in East Kent after 1700, and only eleven for non-nursing 'attending'. These figures may be compared to sixty-four post-1700 references to nursing or nurses' attendance.

In some respects, watching is a comparatively simple service to explain. It involved literally watching someone day and night as a means of monitoring his condition, for the sake of the sick person's comfort and, in some cases, for the safety of those who might be affected by his leaving his bed, whether on account of violence or contagion. Many accounts specify continual 'watching day and night', for instance 'paid to a man and a woman that did continually watche with the said Henry Brodehed in his sicknes by the space of twelve weekes to every of them six pence daye and night'.[63] Most accounts emphasise that the practice of watching was particularly a night-time one, for example 'paid to ij women for watching with David Smithe wyfe deceased one night'.[64] Thus the practice of watching people in their sickness required candles as well as food and drink, 'watching candles' as they are called in one account.[65] However, the subject is not without its methodological complexities. In some instances 'watching' relates to watching with the corpse, prior to burial. This is most commonly found in accounts from Berkshire where men had drowned in the Thames. These state unambiguously that the corpse was watched until the coroner arrived, or until burial.[66] There are no firm indicators that watching took place, as in the old Catholic tradition, as part of a wake. One account notes various gifts to the poor in the medieval style and then has the entry 'paid to the sexton, to the bearers and to widow Foord for "watching"', placing the watching clearly among the funeral items.[67] This account, however, dates to 1644 and thus is almost certainly not an indicator of old Catholic practices dying hard but of watching the man in his sickness. Many accounts include payments for watching along with funeral payments for the reason that very often the women who watched in the time of the sickness also laid out or laid forth the deceased, and/or shrouded him. Other 'watching' contexts could be the watching of a house after the death of the last occupant to safeguard its contents until they could be sold, or the watching of a plague house by a watchman. It is not possible to estimate what the watchers might have done had their subject suddenly taken a turn for the worse: whether they themselves would have acted in a nursing or medical capacity, or whether they would have summoned other help.

[63] PRC 21/8/198.
[64] PRC 2/14/422.
[65] 'Paid to the Physician and Apothecary for their advise & counsell and also for their travell and paynes for and about the said Nicholas and Jone Russell in the tyme of their sicknes wheron [sic] they died and also for meat Drink watching candles and other necessaries in the said time of their sicknes': PRC 2/10/416, dated 1599.
[66] For two cases of watching until the time of burial see BRO, D/A1/195/62a and D/A1/200/101a, transcribed in Berkshire probate accounts, 87, 120 respectively. The earlier of these is a case of death by drowning.
[67] PRC 1/7/5.

Watchers were drawn from the parish community to an even greater extent than attendants generally. Of the thirty-four instances where the parish of a watcher in East Kent is given, only three are not the same as that of the deceased. In one case a poor woman of Faversham was paid for watching a man from Sheppey; it is probable that he fell ill and died in the town.[68] In another case a man from Bridge was paid for watching a man from Kingston, not the adjacent parish but the one beyond.[69] The only other case was of a woman employed to watch with a man from an adjacent parish (Old Romney/Lydd). Dutch communities provided watchers for their members, as may be seen in the entry relating to the congregation in Sandwich: 'paid to Christian Casiar for watching two nights with the sayd Catherine Sciethaze in her sicknes'.[70] But despite this emphasis on the same parish community providing the workforce, there are twenty-one names only partially completed in respect of watching, implying people unfamiliar to the accountant. There are also many references simply to payments for watching, to unnamed individuals. It seems that watching followed the same patterns as non-nursing attendance with regard to the people employed.

Where 'watching' differed from 'attendance' was in the social range of the watchers and the manner of their employment. There is only one reference to a 'Mrs' watching, and no references to anyone of higher social status.[71] Most watchers were paid on a nightly basis, usually at a standard 4d. per night, or on a day-and-night rate, ranging from 4d. to 12d. (normally 6d.). It would appear that the 4d. rate was current as a standard nightly rate through most of the period. Men, it would appear, were usually paid at the higher day-and-night rate of 8d., although a few accounts give equal payments for both sexes.[72] Men were more commonly paid for watching than attending, as a number of early (pre-1640) accounts show. Men, it might be added, only watched for short stints: no account includes a payment for a specific period longer than five nights (although they did 'tend' and act as watchmen for longer periods). Payments to men for watching on a day-and-night basis, or nightly, were rare in respect of contagious illnesses; such payments seem to have been a female preserve. In plague cases long-term watching was often coupled with attendance, thereby linking the two functions as one.

Two accounts demonstrate such points, and the relationship between watching and attending. The first is from the account of Christian Saxten, widow of Ash, with chattels worth £132, whose account is dated 1618:[73]

---

[68] PRC 2/14/494.

[69] PRC 2/8/119.

[70] PRC 2/11/304.

[71] This is 'payde to Goodwife Muncke and Mrs Dadmore for watching with the said decassed in the tyme of his sicknesse': PRC 2/10/395.

[72] For example PRC 21/8/198, which paid the man and woman 6d. each per day and night.

[73] PRC 20/4/360.

Item to certayne wemen for watchinge with the said deceased in the time of her sicknes whereof she dyed, vizt

to Widow Buclland for one night	0s. 4d.
to Goodwyfe Gill for 3 nights and days	1s. 6d.
to Elizabeth Lawrance for 4 nights	2s. 0d.
to Ellen More for 4 days and 3 nights	2s. 0d.
to widdowe Robbins for 4 nights	1s. 4d.

Item to Widdowe Younge of Ashe for her paynes in tendinge of the sayd deceased in the time of her sicknesse whereof she dyed eleven dayes and soe many nights   8s. 0d.

Item for the dyett of the said Widdowe younge for the time of her tendance aforesayd for layinge her forth and for sockinge [the Kentish word for 'shrouding'] her to her buriall   5s 6d.

From these entries it is clear that a series of women might undertake night-time watching duties, and day-and-night watching duties, distinct from the woman who did the 'tendinge'. Only one woman, Widow Young, was paid for attending during this final sickness, compared to five watchers. The total number of nights accounted for is fifteen; the total number of days accounted for is seven; it is possible that the payment to Elizabeth Lawrence for four nights watching should actually read four days (but not necessarily, as periods of night watching often do not equate with days of attendance).[74] Assuming that there is no error, the differing rates of pay in this account for watching and attendance can be determined. Elizabeth Lawrence was paid 6d. per night, compared to the two widows, Buclland and Robbins, who were paid a standard 4d. per night. Goodwife Gill's rate was 6d. per day and night. Ellen More was perhaps paid 6d. per day and night and then 4d. for the extra day. But all these amounts are less than the 8s. paid for Widow Young's tending, which works out at more than 8½ d. per day and night. A similar divergence of responsibilities is to be seen in accounts like that of Robart Sharley, dated 1596, in which three poor women were paid a total of 2s. 'ffor watchinge with the said Robart Sharley in the tyme of his sickenes' but 'Joane tomson' was paid 4s. 'for hyr paynes in attending vpon the said Robarte Sharley in the tyme of his sicknes'.[75]

The second, similarly detailed account, is that of of Robert Legat of Pluckley, who died before 1606 with an estate of just £6:[76]

---

[74] For example, while attending for a week on a sick woman, Goodwife Fearsome only did two nights watching: PRC 2/26/86. Nor was watching always undertaken for the whole period of the illness: see PRC 20/9/319 in which the deceased was ill for ten weeks and yet watching only amounted to 2s. (probably six nights).

[75] PRC 2/8/352.

[76] PRC 2/13/268.

Item paide to George Blackborne for watching with the saide deceased in the tyme of his sicknes whereof hee died   1s. 8d.

Item paide to Goodwyfe Gregorie for watching with the saide deceased in the tyme of his sicknes whereof hee died   0s. 4d.

Item paide and due to be paide to Richard Leggat for watching with the deceassed   1s. 0d.

Item paide to Goodman Man and his wyfe for watching with the said deceassed   3s. 4d.

Item paide and due to be paide to Goodie Tiffell for iij nightes watching with the said deceassed   1s. 0d.

Item paide and due to be paide to Anne Wolfe for watchinge with the deceassed   0s. 4d.

As with the account of Christian Saxten, several watchers were involved, but this was not an excessive number in comparison with some accounts.[77] What is interesting about this account is that no fewer than three of the seven people who watched with the deceased were men, yet there is no sign that this was because of mental derangement or smallpox. Nor is there any payment for attending. It would rather appear that this male accountant (who may have undertaken some attendance himself) chose to employ males as well as females to do the watching.

Further investigation reveals that this bias is borne out generally. Of the seventy-eight instances of men being paid for watching, fifty-seven were cases where the accountant was male compared to twenty-one where the accountant was female. The gender ratio among all carers in all cases of payments for medicine and nursing was 52 per cent male, 48 per cent female. Thus there is some evidence as to how watchers (and by implication attendants) became involved. The next of kin chose people from his circle to act as initial watchers, who then in turn (if the sickness continued) took a role in suggesting other watchers. This explains the instances in the accounts where a watcher's or attendant's name was not fully known to the accountant, indicating that there was little or no prior familiarity with that person, even though they were from the same parish. Through the next of kin, the wider parish community, representing a complex network of friends, kin, close and distant acquaintances, and friends of friends, could be employed as watchers or attenders in cases of protracted ill-health.

To sum up, watching and attendance are often described together, and may in some cases have been interchangeable, there being a degree of cross-over between them, but as service descriptions there are a number of distinctions. Watching was normally undertaken by a series of people, often for

---

[77] A number of late sixteenth- and early seventeenth-century accounts name seven, eight or more helpers and watchers. PRC 21/7/168, dated 1585, records nine different female helpers acting in various roles, from watching to purchasing foodstuffs. PRC 2/3/269, dated 1586, also records nine male and female helpers, including boys and maids, watching and helping.

short stints, and seems to have been paid for on a standard nightly or daily rate. Attendance by comparison was more frequently contracted for at a weekly rate, and structured according to the status of the attendant and the context of the illness. Men undertook watching more often than attendance. Although personnel for both services seem to have been contacted through a chain of personal connections, beginning with the next of kin, watchers were even more frequently drawn from the same parish than attendants. If this is related to the average parish population model, there seems to have been a limited number of semi-occupational experienced women in a parish who attended the dying and were flexible, in that they might perform many essential tasks, from administering necessary broths to washing up linen, for long periods of time. Apart from this group there was a much larger contingent of potential helpers who were able to assist with single tasks less central to the nursing process, from washing (in the case of women) to watching (men or women), probably chosen along the lines of friendship networks and long-term availability more than occupational reputations. There seems to have been little or no remedial expertise (in the context of severe illnesses) associated with this group. If the average attendant was not expected to have significantly more medical knowledge than the average married woman, then the average watcher was not expected to have any more medical or health-related experience than the average boy or girl. With respect to this last assertion the account of Tobyas Odley, dated 1585, includes the entry 'paid to a boy for ii nightes watchynge with the said Tobyas odley in his sicknes'.[78]

Nursing

The term 'nursing' is as multi-faceted today as it was at the end of the seventeenth century, and is still not one which can be defined exclusively by occupation. Modern arguments about the health-related roles of carers in the home and in institutions require the word to have both broad and narrow meanings, ranging from the remedial to simple assistance in lifting and steadying, and to mean different things in different contexts. It is reasonable to suppose that over the period 1660–1720 the word had, or was then developing, a similarly complex series of meanings. However, the starting point must be actual instances of the word being used. From these it is possible to move on to other, less clear, meanings and implications.

An account dated 1667 has the entry 'paid unto Lamentus Simms widow who was put in as a nurse to attend the said deceased a little before she died and for the time she remained there afterwards for the cleaning and airing of the goods'.[79] Such an entry is a suitable place at which to begin as it indicates two things. First, by stating that this woman was acting 'as a nurse' it suggests

[78] PRC 2/3/269.
[79] PRC 1/12/96.

163

that the role of a nurse was established, and widely understood, but that this particular woman was only acting in this capacity: it did not constitute a normal part of her identity. Second, it indicates that the main function of a nurse was attendance. Although she also cleaned and aired the goods afterwards, these functions are distinguished from her nursing role. There are five other entries which similarly describe women acting 'as a nurse', and all these also give 'attendance' and 'looking after' as the key nursing functions.[80]

These entries raise an important question. If a nurse was also 'tending' and 'looking after' what, if anything, distinguished her from the non-nursing attendants? One answer to this has already been given: date, nursing being largely a feature of post-Restoration accounts. But more important are the discernible aspects of nurses' identities. Only women were described as 'nurses'. Perhaps the old understanding of wet-nursing extended into the early seventeenth century, and thus carried the association of 'nursing' with exclusively female care, but it is noticeable that no male is referred to in these accounts as a 'nurse'. This is not to say that men were never paid for 'nursing', but where they were, they were paid for providing nursing, such as 'paid Robert Elvy as per bill for nursing and about the funeral',[81] and 'paid to John Moore for nurses and looking after the said deceased and his family ... they being sick of the smallpox'.[82] Some cases are ambiguous: the medical practitioner named might have been providing nurses but more probably was simply mentioned in an entry which concatenated payments to the practitioner and for nursing assistance.[83] There is only one payment to a man personally for 'nursing' in all these accounts: 'paid to Thomas Hatch for likewise lookeing to or Nurseing of the said deceased in his said last sicknes'.[84] And even the writer of this singular example was doubtful whether Thomas Hatch's service should be described as nursing.

The exclusivity of the words 'nurse' and 'nursing' in East Kent may be explored further. Unsurprisingly, there are no boys described as nurses. There are no references to 'maids' acting in this capacity either. In fact the last reference to a maid or maid-servant being paid for attending or watching (even in a non-nursing capacity) was in the 1640s; after the Restoration they were only mentioned when the patient died in other people's houses and the servants were paid for their trouble. One account from 1666 sepa-

---

[80] These are PRC 2/35/252, dated 1674; PRC 2/38/148, dated 1679; PRC 2/40/185, dated 1684; PRC 20/13/541, dated 1685; and PRC 1/16/10, dated 1698.
[81] PRC 1/16/73.
[82] PRC 1/17/43, dated 1711. This is one of only a very few references to a man 'for nurses'; it need not mean that he provided them, but rather that he had undertaken to pay them.
[83] For example, 'paid unto Mr Golder phisitian for phisick administred to the said deceased in his sicknes whd and for attendance of nurses in that sicknes in all': PRC 20/12/283; or 'paid vnto Dr Dade & Mr Taylor for phisick by them administred to the said deceased in the time of her sickness ... & for the attendance of Nurses': PRC 2/36/117.
[84] PRC 20/12/108, dated 1674

rates the two roles: 'paid to the deceased's maid servant for wages and to a nurse for her attendance on the said deceased in her sickness and for socking and laying her forth'.[85] Another striking aspect of nursing identities is that no woman was described as both a midwife and a nurse except in a childbirth context. In such instances a midwife might be paid for attending a woman 'in her sickness'.[86] As Margaret Pelling has pointed out, references to midwives 'do not often lead one to nurses, of any kind'.[87] In 1618 Cicely Gittins acted as a midwife and as a watcher to the same family, but this is the only case in the East Kent accounts where a known midwife was given the identity of a bedside attendant.[88] In the account of John Clay (1608) a nurse and a midwife were paid together for attending a man and his wife; the fact that they were given different occupational identities when they were both 'attending' only reinforces the impression that it was usual to draw a hard and fast distinction between midwives and other attendants, including nurses.[89] A last clear difference between 'nursing' and other attendance is that nurses were hardly ever described as poor. There is only one such reference, an early one, dated 1609.[90]

Such identity boundaries indicate that the descriptive terms 'nurse' and 'nursing' were relatively exclusive in sick-nursing contexts, at least after 1660. This raises the question of whether the women so described were more specifically sought-after, and sought from further afield, and thus perhaps less well-known to the deceased and his next of kin than the general attenders from the wider parish community. Unfortunately there is insufficient data on this matter. Only one 'nurse' has been noted as being partially named, with a blank left for her Christian name, but women described as nurses were less regularly named than those who were not.[91] The same lack of definition appears in respect to hometowns: very few nurses' places of residence are given. Thus it is much harder to establish whether these were women from the local parish community. It may be that the very lack of names is an indicator of unfamiliarity, but it would be unwise to assume this without further evidence.

[85] PRC 1/12/48.
[86] For example, 'paid to Goodwife Mason the midwiffe for attending on the said Mary in her sicknes': PRC 21/6/263, dated 1583.
[87] Pelling, Common lot, 182.
[88] PRC 2/22/104. It should be noted, however, that there are instances of nurses paid for acting in childbirth scenarios, such as 'paid to Nurse Cox for tending the said deceased in the time of his last sickness and for keeping the said deceased's widow in the time of her lying-in of child birth': PRC 1/9/28, dated 1662.
[89] PRC 2/14/110.
[90] PRC 2/13/247.
[91] 'Paid to [blank] West for nursing the deceased in his last sickness': PRC 19/6/66, dated 1717. Another example, which seems clearly to indicate a nurse otherwise unknown to the accountant, is 'paid to one Lame a nurse who attended the said intestate in her sicknes whereof he dyed': PRC 2/41/81. Less than 20% of 'nurses' are named compared to about 30% of attenders and watchers, and there are many fewer specified 'nurses'.

Another opportunity to test how sought-after nurses were by comparison with other attendants is by means of a comparison of the wages paid, and the types of contract that they might have agreed. In this respect the most valuable accounts are those in which nurses and other attendants appear. There are only a few of these. One is the 1622 account of Peter Bull, in which Goodwife Browne was paid 6s. 'for her paines in attending the said deceased' and Nurse Whitfeild was paid 30s. for the same.[92] In this instance it is not clear how many weeks each woman served, nor what they actually did. A nurse seems to be paid at a separate rate in the 1674 account of David Russell of Cranbrook, in which Goodwife Boreman was paid 30s. for six weeks' attendance 'as a Nurse' and Mary Marten was paid 8s. for two weeks 'attendance'.[93] Hence the woman explicitly described as a nurse was paid 5s. per week compared to the other woman's 4s. But it could be argued that payments among non-nurses varied at least to this extent, and therefore too much should not be read into the difference.

A systematic comparison of remuneration for nursing and non-nursing attendance reveals very similar wage levels. Those cases where rates were specified, and were thus probably contractual, show that attendance on plague and smallpox victims normally merited regular payments of 7s.–10s. per week in both nursing or non-nursing contexts. Nursing rates otherwise could be as low as 2s. 6d. and 3s. per week: as low as the lowest non-nursing attendance rates other than those to the poor. Averaging all the weekly rates reveals that nursing was, at approximately 6.1s. per week (1642–1700), not much better paid than attendance at 5.3s. per week (1578–1696). If the references to payments of 1s. 6d. and less, which seem to relate to payments to the poor for attending are discounted, then the average rate for non-nursing attendance is 6.1s. per week, exactly the same as nursing. It could be hypothesised that nursing and attendance were effectively the same service, except that the poor and inexperienced were not described as nurses.

The problem is that the amounts themselves do not reveal the nature or length of service prior to the last period of attendance. It could be that references to nursing relate to a greater proportion of longer, more drawn-out relationships between a patient and 'his nurse'. There are instances in which nurses were described possessively, just as occasionally physicians were linked to 'their' patients. For instance one 1667 account records a payment 'unto Elizabeth Mitchener the said deceased's nurse for her attendance upon the said deceased ... she dying of the smallpox'.[94] The 1682 account of George Petts records a payment 'to a woman who attended on the said deceased in that sicknes as his nurse 10s.'.[95] In the same year the account of Richard Bradshaw notes a sum of 10s. paid to 'the woman who attended on the

92 PRC 2/23/30.
93 PRC 2/35/252.
94 PRC 1/12/54.
95 PRC 20/13/186.

Table 61
Payments in respect of attendance, in nursing and non-nursing contexts

	Mean total payments for 'nursing' and 'attendance' by nurses (not in conjunction with other services)	Mean total payments for non-nursing 'attendance' incl. 'looking after/to' (not in conjunction with other services)
1570–89	–	4s. 3d.
1590–9	–	11s. 3d.
1600–9	[7s. 0d.]	7s. 2d.
1610–19	[10s.]	10s. 2 d.
1620–9	[19s. 6d.]	14s. 4d.
1630–9	[280s.]	17s. 2d.
1640–9	[16s. 8d.]	21s. 4d.
1660–9	48s. 3d.	35s. 7d.
1670–9	27s. 7d.	21s. 5d.
1680–9	22s. 6d.	15s. 0d.
1690–9	19s. 4d.	14s. 6d.
1700–9	16s. 5d.	[5s. 4d.]
1710–19	24s. 1d.	[5s. 2d.]

Note: Figures in square brackets are based on fewer than ten separate payments. The 1630–9 payment of 280s. is an isolated payment.

said deceased in his sicknes of which he dyed as his nurse'.[96] There are no equivalent possessive references to non-nursing attendants or watchers. What seems to be reflected in these entries is a relationship, which, as with physicians, very probably relates to a bond of trust between the patient and 'his' nurse. Time was probably a critical factor in allowing such a bond to develop. If average rates for nursing and attending were equal, and largely static across the period, it is difficult to see how average payments for nursing after 1660 could have been invariably higher than attendance unless they related to longer periods of service.

Given the similarity between contract-type rates for nursing attendance and general attendance, it is reasonable to suppose that many women who could have been described as nurses (but who were not) appear in the 'non-nursing' column in table 61. Despite this, for the period during which nursing was common (after 1660), payments for general attendance were consistently between two-thirds and three-quarters of the payments for nursing or attendance by nurses. This leads to the supposition that it is probably not discrepancies but similarities between nursing and other contractual attend-

[96] PRC 19/4/106. Likewise Mary Ellis was paid 12s. in 1714 for attending on John Whiting 'as his nurse': PRC 1/17/65; and Goodwife Cuttbush was described in 1712 as 'the said deceased's nurse': PRC 1/17/47.

ance that should be sought in this period. Instances in which experienced females were paid for long stints at a set rate have more in common with the functions of nurses than with nondescript persons who performed stints of watching on a nightly basis.

Very few nurses' names appear more than once in the accounts, and so it is not possible to rebuild their practices. However, some key evidence does emerge. It is significant that there are more cases of names repeated in separate accounts in the period after 1660 than before (Nurse Alcock is the only certain case before 1650, despite 70 per cent of accounts predating the Interregnum). This suggests that nursing (broadly defined) may have been a more regular occupation for those who practised it after the Restoration. In 1674 Goodwife Booreman was paid 30s. for six weeks' attendance 'as a nurse' on a Cranbrook man, and ten years later, as Widow Booreman, she was paid 5s. for attending John Chandler in Biddenden, the neighbouring parish.[97] In Sandwich, in the 1660s, Mary Dods was twice called upon to 'attend' a house struck with plague, being paid at the rate of 8s. 6d. per week.[98] In 1662 Goodwife Fuller 'the deceased's nurse' was paid for 'attending on and looking to the said deceased in the time of his sickness', and it seems likely that, three years later, as Widow Fuller, she was paid for 'nursing the said deceased's wife and child' in a multiple infection case in a neighbouring parish.[99] But the most interesting two individuals to be named more than once in these accounts are Widow Grant of the Thanet region in the 1690s, and Widow Riall of Ospringe in the period 1681–1712. Widow Grant is the only woman identified in these accounts as undertaking a nursing role in respect of one dying patient (of St John's Thanet) and a medical one in respect of the child of another (of Monkton), whose sore leg she healed.[100] The two other payments which hint at nurses possibly administering physic are ambiguously worded, but these may also support the possibility that nurses in some circumstances might themselves oversee a medical treatment.[101] In this sense they may have been performing much the same function as the next of kin, obtaining well-known medicines from an apothecary to administer to the sick or dying person. Finally, there is the case of Widow Riall, who is first encountered in an account from Ospringe dated 1681, in which she was paid for watching with a dying yeoman.[102] Three years later she appears as 'the widow Riall ... for her attendance and nurshing the said deceased and his wife in the time of their sicknes whereof they dyed and

[97] PRC 2/35/252, PRC 2/40/185.
[98] PRC 1/14/37, PRC 1/12/8.
[99] PRC 1/11/41, PRC 1/9/50.
[100] PRC 2/42/5, PRC 19/5/15.
[101] These both date from 1672: 'for the funerall ... and for the Nurses that attended him in his sickness whereof he died and for Physick then administred unto him': PRC 2/35/147; and 'paid vnto the Nurses that did tend and watch with the said deceased in his sicknes whereof he dyed and for physicke then administred to him': PRC 2/35/104.
[102] PRC 2/39/162.

... for necessaryes for them in that time'.[103] She is also possibly the Widow Riall, also described as 'Nurce Royal', who tended another couple who died together, in Luddenham (two parishes from Ospringe), in a 1712 account. Although there was no medical element to what Widow Riall was doing (as far as can be established), she was in four instances attending and looking after, and in two of these four she is either described as a nurse or paid for nursing. If it is correct to identify all four references as relating to the same woman, it is also clear that women of her experience might travel between parishes and retain the identities of both widow and nurse.

On this basis arguments on nursing and non-nursing attendance after 1660 may be strengthened. The former was without doubt a more specialist or experienced subset of the latter, defined in part by the exclusivity of the terminology which discounted men, the poor, occasional short-term helpers and the inexperienced from being referred to as nurses, and in part by the nature of nursing contracts, which effectively meant that a woman should attend a patient for as long as necessary at an agreed fixed rate. Judging from the evidence relating to contractual 'attendants', it is very likely that most nurses were drawn from the wider parish community (not kin and direct friends), including secondary contacts from adjacent parishes and perhaps the parish beyond that. After the Interregnum period the trend seems to have been for palliative assistance increasingly to have been described in this way; thus the cadre of occupational or semi-occupational female attendants in each parish who were the most versatile and flexible 'attendants' in the pre-1650 period seem to have received an identity and a descriptor in the term 'nurse'. The widespread use of this word after 1660 allows for confidence in stating that the occupational or semi-occupational sick-nurse was definitely a feature of the East Kent socio-economic landscape by 1660. Paid local non-'nursing' help, including 'watching', seems to have all but disappeared by about 1710. By 1700 most paid attendance was understood to be the prerogative of occupational or semi-occupational 'nurses'.

If the temporal boundary is extended to 1730 the ideal nurse is seen in Thomas Fuller's list of requirements, as expressed in his book on eruptive fevers (especially measles and smallpox).[104] Fuller assumes that a nurse is female, and stresses the desirability of her being (among other things) middle-aged, healthy, a good watcher, with good hearing and sight, nimble, cleanly, cheerful, sober, without dependent children and that she be 'observant to follow the Physicians Orders duly; and not be so conceited of her own Skill as to give her own medicines privately'. While it is impossible to know whether East Kent nurses were cleanly, nimble and cheerful, or even sober, they were often paid alongside physicians and surgeons, they tended to be more expe-

---

[103] PRC 2/40/191.
[104] T. Fuller, *Exanthematologia: or, an attempt to give a rational account of eruptive fevers, especially of the measles and small pox*, London 1730, quoted in Bullough and Bullough, *Care of the sick*, 57.

rienced women, and they might travel across a couple of parishes to attend a dying person (suggesting that they were sought-after). Lastly, Fuller's intimation that they might have sufficient confidence in their medical skills to undertake a cure (in the context of 'eruptive fevers') may well support the suggestion, already advanced, that there was a medical element to nursing contagious diseases.

This broad outline of the development of nursing presents two paradoxes. The first is that paid nursing was increasing in volume at a time when large sections of the potential workforce (for example the poor, men, boys and maids) were increasingly being excluded from the caring industry. A second lies in the fact that, as this more exclusive 'nursing' was taking over as the dominant form of palliative care, and the workforce was becoming arguably more feminised and experienced, the average amounts paid to nurses and similar attendants dropped very significantly. These two features appear to run contrary to the basic demand and supply laws of economics. However, the second paradox is simple to explain: the disease landscape changed. Plague, which had been such an important cause of long-term nursing and attendance, ceased to play a part in people's lives and deaths. Payments in respect of plague nursing escalated over the course of the seventeenth century, from an average of about 28s. in 1610–19 to 98s. 6d. in 1660–9. These large payments did not cease overnight, as some accounts were not submitted until ten or more years after the last plague cases (five accounts for plague victims with nursing entries date from the 1670s, one from as late as 1679). The high payments for smallpox nursing also tail off, predominantly dating from the 1670s (54s. average) and 1680s (46s. average). Thus the descending figures in table 62 do not show nursing and attendance being valued less highly than in previous years, but purchased more often for short periods of time, or less often for long periods of time, and less frequently in the context of particularly feared illnesses such as plague and smallpox. Although it is impossible to exclude contagious diseases entirely from an estimate of payments in respect of nursing, it is clear that the overall drop in the average amounts paid for nursing is not as dire as appeared in the previous table.

The other paradox – that overall levels of nursing care increased as the workforce became more narrowly focused – is interesting as it may be seen to be contemporary with (and similar to) the greater provision of medical help by a cohort of male practitioners which was not growing larger and may have been shrinking in size. With regard to the latter this was possibly partly due to the relocation of practitioners in rural areas and to the greater availability and transportability of medicines. Neither explanation can apply to nurses, as they were probably already close to their patients through residence in the same or adjacent parishes. But the obvious parallel to draw is that of specialisation, or division of labour. Medical practitioners were increasingly facilitating medical provision by concentrating on providing medicines as well as acting as surgeons, and taking on new roles beyond the limits of their

Table 62
Total value of payments for nursing and other 'attendance'
excluding plague, smallpox, 'visitations' etc.

	Nursing attendance	Other attendance
1660–9	22s. 6d.	24s. 10d.
1670–9	25s. 6d.	20s. 4d.
1680–9	20s. 1d.	13s. 11d.
1690–9	16s. 0d.	15s. 2d.
1700–19	16s. 7d.	[5s. 7d.]

Note: Figures in square brackets are based on fewer than ten separate payments.

official qualifications, thereby effectively becoming full-time general practitioners. Women were doing something similar: 'specialising' (in the sense of
providing a range of specialist skills) and taking on wider roles (including
possibly administering medicine in some instances, as well as attending and
watching). It is probably no coincidence that the exclusively female word
'nurse' became dominant in the diocese of Canterbury at the same time as
the exclusively male word 'doctor' became the most common way to describe
male practitioners.

'Keeping', 'helping', 'work' and 'boarding'

In any exploration of nursing in the early modern period it is important to
understand the variations of – and the ambiguities in – the language used.
This entails examining not just the contextual variations of obvious words
such as 'attendance' and 'nurse' but the incidental meanings of other relevant
words, and their contextual variations. The two most important examples
are 'helping' and 'keeping'; 'work' and 'boarding' may also be added. These
words have meanings so wide and general that they are frequently to be
found in the East Kent accounts, and although in many cases they were not
meant to imply nursing or medical help, in other cases they certainly were.

In 'Nurses and nursekeepers' Pelling stresses the importance of the words
'keeping' and 'helping', stating that it is within these terms 'that the activity
of nursing may be found'.[105] This statement was made in the context of iden-
tifying women's occupations in the late sixteenth-century Norwich 'census',
but it could also relate to late sixteenth-century Kent probate accounts. The
word 'keeping' especially is found in contexts which relate to the provision
of sustenance and cleaning of the sick and dying. 'Paid to Sases wydow for
kepinge of the testatrix in the tyme of her sicknes' is a not uncommon

[105] Pelling, *Common lot*, 194.

171

payment formula.[106] Undoubtedly in East Kent the word covers nursing activity too. But given the broad range of functions a 'keeper' might undertake, it is questionable how often it relates to nursing activities. The word in every instance may be taken to mean feeding, but it does not in every instance also mean the purchasing and taking home of provisions, watching, attending, cleaning, washing, restraining and administering medicine to the sick person. Sometimes it is clear that there are boundaries, and that the word does not automatically include a certain function, especially when that function is otherwise described. The phrase 'paid unto a woman that kept and watched with the said Margarett whyles she lay sick' suggests that 'watching' was construed to be additional to, and not part of, 'keeping' and therefore required separate specification.[107] This applies to 'tending' too, as in 'for the kepinge of James Cock by the space of 16 dayes and for watching and tending of hym being sick'.[108] It also applies to the fetching of physic, and cleaning.[109] All these references date from the late sixteenth century. Keeping a dependent person fed and watered and (cleanly) evacuated are probably the only functions that may be assumed always to be implicit in 'keeping' references in these accounts. The role of the 'keeper' was an expandable one, which involved feeding and a number of other things as and when they might have become necessary. It did not necessarily even relate to illness, as 'keeping' a dependent child did not require that child to be ill. Almost the only certainty is that 'keeping' in East Kent was on the decline as a description of nursing services by 1610 and defunct by 1660. Given that 'nursing' references are common only after this latter date, it might reasonably be supposed that 'keeping' was another expression of nursing activities, just a much more general one.

The general applications of the word 'keeping' may explain why it appears in a census-like document, such as that for Norwich. It was a catch-all term, applicable to a sufficiently large body of women for it to have collective meaning. In the late sixteenth century it might be said that 'attendants' were a subset of 'keepers' in much the same way that 'watchers' were subsets of 'attendants'. But this generality does not help the historian who is trying to establish the medical knowledge required of a 'keeper'. To what extent did feeding a person involve treatment? If the food was diet drinks and broths, then probably there was a considerable treatment element. If not, the oppo-

---

[106] PRC 21/3/254, dated 1577.

[107] PRC 21/2/253. Other examples include PRC 21/4/190, PRC 21/6/405, PRC 2/5/51, PRC 2/11/304, PRC 21/7/168 and many others.

[108] PRC21/6/272. Other examples include PRC 2/11/294, PRC 2/12/11, PRC 2/12/418, PRC 2/15/101 and many others.

[109] 'Paid to suche as kepte the said John Clercke in the tyme of his sicknes beeing a long tyme for phisick and other necessarie thinges fet [sic] for him in his sicknes and owing at his death': PRC 2/6/71; 'paide to certen women that kepte the saide deceassed in her sicknes & for washing the clothes woollen & lynnen of the said deceassed': PRC 2/10/114.

site view might be taken. The important point is that, either way, a person was being paid to provide a necessary function, to help those incapable of feeding themselves. This is a clear necessity of nursing. But to apply such a definition of nursing to the interpretation of a probate account is the equivalent of including as a 'nurse' the person who was paid for obtaining or providing a meal, or perhaps someone who cooked that meal to order. Both activities might affect the health of the patient but neither necessarily relates to therapeutic knowledge. Although Margaret Pelling has shown that attitudes to diet as a function of preserving health and treating ill-health were common, and not the preserve of physicians, the preparation of food was not synonymous with medical assistance.[110] Even if all 'keeping' is related to the cadre of experienced and versatile local women in each parish, it would be rash to presume that a payment to a 'keeper' necessarily implies that there was any greater medical emphasis in what the patient was fed in the last days of his life. The generality of the word thus undermines attempts to interpret its medical relevance without further context. After all, one could be a good 'keeper' without the patient being sick at all (for example the young or very old). This contrasts with 'attendance' and 'tending', where there was an added specific obligation to observe and help with the malady from which the patient was suffering. Thus 'keeping', when it appears in the probate accounts, should be construed as relating to nursing but often only of the most general kind and not necessarily involving medical knowledge.

There is one sense in which the 'keeping' function was very definitely an activity with a clear health-related element. This is when a sick patient was deliberately taken into a house to be tended as well as kept. Obviously this is different from situations in which the deceased happened to fall ill in someone else's house and remained there, kept, until he died, but it is often very difficult to be sure from the accounts which type of attendance away from home is meant, whether the patient was deliberately taken to a house to be nursed, or just fell ill and died while visiting someone's house. Since the vast majority of people in these accounts died at home, examples of both types are a small minority, the former being the rarer of the two. Some examples occur in relation to medical help, such as 'paid for the chardges of the said Richard [from Rainham] lienge [lying] at Maydston duringe the time that the said Richard Trierst was under the Cures of the said Mr Bennet'.[111] Others do not, for example 'paid ... to three men for carrying the said Robert Coppin from the waterside to the howse of wydowe waters where hee dyed the said deceassd beeing taken sicke on the water'.[112] In most instances the practice of looking after individuals in a house other than their own is

110 Pelling, *Common lot*, 40.
111 PRC 2/10/311, dated 1599.
112 PRC 20/2/27, dated 1609. In this case 'wydowe waters' was also paid 'for fruite and spices and ... for other victualls bowght for and spent by the said deceased in the tyme of his sicknes whereof hee dyed'.

not described as 'keeping' but 'boarding and dieting' or 'lodging'. The prime examples of this sort of keeping are those few sad cases in which a disease had taken over someone's life so completely that it had caused them to leave their home and spend sums of money well beyond their means in trying to obtain a cure. The account, dated 1674, of Catherine Symons of Sandwich is one such:[113]

Item paid vnto John Smith ... for the said deceaseds board from the 29th of September 1667 to the 12th of April 1668	£7
Item paid unto Isaac Peirs ... for her board from the 12th of April 1668 to the 29th of September next following	£4 16s.
Item paid vnto Gabriel Adams ... for her board from the 29th of September 1668 to the 27th of April next following	£6
Item paid for removing the said deceased from Sandwich to Denton with the trunke 10s., and vnto Mr Boughton the phisitian for phisicke administred to her while she was att Denton 40s., and for a woman to attend there (she having a Cancer in her stomach of which she dyed as was sayed by her severall phisitians) 10s.	£3
Item paid for the removing the said deceased from Denton to Canterbury 7s., and for a weekes board & attendance there to Mr Cox 8s., and unto Mr Peters for phisick and attendance on her in that time 10s.	25s.
Item paid for the removing the said deceased from Canterbury to Sandwich with her trunke 7s., and vnto Mr Isaac Peirs for her board from the first day of May 1669 to the 29th of September 1669 £4 8s., and paid unto him for phisick for the said deceased in that time 25s. 6d., & for a woman's attendance 7s. 6d.	£6 8s.
Item paid for the removing the said deceased from Sandwich to Eythorne with her trunke 5s., and to Roger Castle for her board there from the 29th of September 1669 to the 17th of January following £3 4s.	£3 9s.
Item paid for the removing the said deceased from Eythorne to John Brownes of Sandwich 3s., and vnto the said John Browne for her board & lodging from the 17th day of January 1669 to the 17th of October next following the summe of Ten pounds during which time she lay [in] such great extremity of paine by rason of her aforesaid distemper that none could endure the roome but upon great necessity £10	£10 3s.
Item paid vnto the Nurses that attended the said deceased in that her sicknes att the aforesaid John Brownes house and for <laying> her forth when she dyed	£1 15s.

[113] PRC 2/36/123. Note that the chronology of this case might be confused. Isaac Peirs (d.1706) was a surgeon of Eythorne; thus the payments to him for boarding and physic might be incorrectly associated with Sandwich in the account.

This account clearly shows that Catherine stayed in a house run by a surgeon assisting her as well as houses of non-practitioners who were merely looking after her while she was attended by other people. In all these cases an atmosphere of hoped-for recovery can be expected to have prevailed, and thus there is no good reason to suppose there was a greater medical element to her boarding in Isaac Peirs's house than in, say, that of Mr Cox. Where there are payments for boarding in other people's houses, it cannot be assumed that the reason was accidental rather than remedial, even where these were not the houses of practitioners.

In conclusion, in records which describe co-operation and support in chronic disease and other end-of-life contexts, it is very difficult to draw a line between routine and special help. Everyday support shades gradually into palliative care, which in turn shades gradually into the active attendance of experienced nurses, and ultimately medical care. Along this medical spectrum may be placed ranges of language, so that a broad spectrum of non-medical to palliative care is covered by a word such as 'boarding and dieting', and an even broader range is covered by 'keeping', including the subset 'attendance' at the medical end of this range, and 'nursing' reaching even further up the medical scale. 'Work' is probably to be placed low on the medical scale, and although covering a broad range (as it can cover many household functions), being relatively impersonal it is a term rarely used in the context of attendance. All these terms overlap and inter-relate, and to remove any one of them from the vocabulary of nursing would be to distort the range of activities undertaken. Hence this study, by applying a cautious – perhaps exclusive – definition to nursing services, has narrowed the range. Having said that, the evidence from an exclusive definition of nursing services suggests that the development of nursing noted with regard to sick-nursing in chapter 1 is reflected in changes in the nature of those services. As sick-nursing declined as an activity carried out in isolation from paid medical intervention so it became not so much a series of activities carried out by the community in general but increasingly the province of the 'nurse', who was drawn from a small part of the community: experienced women without young children.

Nurses, responsibility and the medical initiative

The bulk of nursing services can thus be arranged in an overlapping series of ranges between notional boundaries: one extreme verging on medical assistance; the other non-nursing 'work'. Thus it is a two-dimensional mapping of the range of sick-nursing services. It could be argued that this excludes aspects of nursing included in a multi-dimensional approach, such as that put forward by Margaret Pelling. However, for quantitative purposes this is impossible to use, as it is too general to measure. Instead a simplification might be considered: a nurse who attended the dying might have had an

Table 63
Direction of medical strategies in East Kent

	1570–1609 %	1610–49 %	1660–89 %	1690–1719 %
Accounts which record medical practitioners whose first-hand advice was or may have been given (practitioner-directed strategies)	14–26	21–48	61–80	76–87
Accounts which record nursing assistance but no medical practitioners or medical advice (home- or nursing-directed strategies)	73–9	49–62	18–25	10–12
Accounts which record only purchases of medicines and no medical advice nor nursing care (home-directed strategies)	1–6	3–16	2–13	3–12

occasional medical role in parallel with her nursing one. This begs the question: who was directing the care strategy if a nurse was employed but no medical practitioner? Conclusions to date have been derived from records of consumption, and the implicit assumption that whoever was footing the bill – the family of the deceased – was responsible for directing the care strategy has not been seriously questioned. Where medical practitioners were called in to advise the victim and family, then it might reasonably be assumed that the direction of the care strategy had, in whole or in part, been delegated, at least temporarily, to that practitioner. To what extent, therefore, might responsibility for the care strategy have been delegated to attendants, nurses, keepers and other helpers?

In pursuing this line of enquiry it is necessary to consider the relative roles of three groups: family (including household), experienced attendants and medical advisers; medical advisers must be separated out from medical practitioners. Possible levels of responsibility are set out in table 63.[114]

If it is assumed that the midpoint in each range is representative, then it seems that medical advice was purchased in only 20 per cent of care strategies in the early period but in about 80 per cent in the last. The average attendant and watcher or keeper seems to have been employed for services more closely resembling a household servant model rather than a medical one, especially in the early decades. Thus it would be highly unwise to use the decline in employment of attendants compared to physicians as a measurement of the decline of attendants' authority over their patients. But it is reasonable to suppose that such a dramatic rise in the level of medical advice

---

[114] For an explanation of why the figures in table 63 are ranges see Mortimer, 'Medical assistance', i. 308; ii. 154.

Table 64
Nursing practitioners' independent payments for medicines in East Kent

	1570– 1609 %	1610– 49 %	1660– 89 %	1690– 1719 %
Accounts which record nursing but no medical advice	73–79	49–62	18–25	10–12
Accounts which record payments for medicines independently of medical advisers as a % of the above	2–11	3–27	3–39	3–28

Note: The lower row is calculated as a percentage of the midpoint in the range of the upper row.

given by practitioners resulted in a diminution in the control of care strategies by nurses and attendants. Thus the value of establishing the maximum possible level of control exercised by nurses and attendants in table 63 is not so much to assess the level itself as to establish the level of medicinal purchases which were undertaken by nurses independent of physicians and surgeons.

As the proportion of care strategies directed by medical practitioners increased, so too did the number of cases in which medicines were perhaps purchased by nurses (*see* table 64). It seems that, while nurses' control over care strategies diminished, the proportion of nurses who took a medical initiative in purchasing medicines increased, with the result that nurses and attendants acting independently of medical practitioners were responsible for purchasing a small but significant proportion (perhaps about 5–15 per cent) of all medicines bought on behalf of dying patients for whom accounts survive.

This analysis supports earlier impressions of nursing and attendance. In the early period most care was provided by the family and household and, where assistance was sought, it was sought from the wider parish community largely for the purposes of help within the house. A small number of assistants were more experienced and able to take an appropriate medical initiative. In the early seventeenth century the terminology began to change, and nurses found themselves more frequently working alongside medical practitioners, more exclusively employed as semi-occupational 'nurses' but directing care strategies less regularly. By 1700 the frequency with which casual household helpers were employed had diminished practically to zero, and nursing had become a recognised occupation, with an identity and set of expectations of those in the role. One of those expectations may well have been an ability in emergencies and extreme cases to take medical action independently; this may account for the small but significant level of medicinal expenditure which may be associated with nurses attending the dying.

Subsidiary services

Discussion of the nursing services reflected in the probate accounts cannot fail to mention several services which are frequently described and which are directly or indirectly related to nursing. 'Keeping', of course, involved the regular use of attendance for fetching things, especially food, for the deceased. Equally frequently mention is made of 'cleaning' performed by attendants. The role of attendants and nurses in funeral arrangements is also obviously a common feature of these accounts. All of these services require comment for they all impact on the attendants' roles.

A 1648 reference quoted in 'Nurses and nursekeepers' describes the nurse's role as that of 'dressing meat, keeping clean the clothes of the infected people, and cleansing and making habitable their houses'.[115] A century earlier, the refounding of St Bartholomew's Hospital, London, had provided for a matron and her 'sisters' to make beds and to 'wash and attend upon the said poor men and women there'.[116] Should each separate part of this conglomeration of nursing services be regarded as an element of nursing? There are many payments for fetching or purchasing specific items in the Kent accounts, and certain of them, through their regularity in fatal disease contexts, suggest a therapeutic – or at least traditional or ritual – course of action. For example, chickens and mutton were very regularly purchased on behalf of the dying: 'for two neckes of mutton and other thinges provided for the said deceased in the time of his last sickness' being the usual expression.[117] The large number of references to mutton in particular point to those nursed at home being fed much the same diet as those in early hospitals.[118] References to mutton and chickens are often combined with payments for spices and fruit, including plums, prunes, sugar, currants, raisins, almonds, nutmeg and ginger. Contexts for such entries make it clear that these are for the benefit of the sick person, not those attending them, for example 'laid out by this accomptant out of his owne purse for plumes sugar wyne Candles mutton and other such like necessaries and nutryments for the deceased testator in the time of his sicknes whereof he died and which was never repaid' or 'for syrops, conserves, 1 lb sugar, 2 lb prunes, ½lb almonds, nutmeg and ginger, mutton, a chick, coles, candles, aquavite, 3 quartes of sacke, a pint of muskveen, a quart of white wine and ale'.[119] In both these entries are seen most of the makings (minus the eggs and gruel) of caudled ale – a special broth for use in nursing treatments – or spiced wine. Great attention was paid to diet in

[115] Pelling, *Common lot*, 197. This was in respect of attending plague victims in Middlewich (Cheshire), and merited a remuneration of 7s. plus diet.
[116] Quoted in Bullough and Bullough, *Care of the sick*, 55.
[117] PRC 2/34/67.
[118] Bullough and Bullough, *Care of the sick*, 59.
[119] PRC 20/7/106, dated 1626; PRC 2/3/263, dated 1586.

the cases reflected in these accounts; hence 'dieting' references most probably should be understood in a more medical light than at first strikes the modern reader.[120] This is especially so in the sixteenth century, when the importance of diet was valued knowledge, and spices might be obtained from an apothecary as well as a grocer.[121] Although, as with so many non-nursing entries, the majority of payments in respect of mutton, lamb, chickens and spices predate 1650, it would be wrong to presume that diet lost importance, especially as such payments might have become subsumed within payments for nursing. Also some late payments explicitly mention these foodstuffs in nursing contexts, such as 'for meate, fruite, spices and attendance on the said deceased in his sickness' in an account dated 1665.[122] 'For a neck of mutton in her illness' appears in an account dated 1712.[123] From this it can be said that the references to 'keeping', which were counted as an estimate of nursing provision in the tables in chapter 1, should be supplemented in regard to the provision of foodstuffs, but to what extent this should equate to an amplification of the nursing services generally it is not possible to say.

Cleaning was certainly a function very frequently undertaken by attendants and nurses, but again it is debatable how much 'cleaning' by itself should be regarded as an indicator of nursing. While many accounts show the cleaning in an unambiguous nursing context, for example 'Fyrst payd and layd oute unto Trenchemes wyfe for watching and washing with the said Bennett Daye in the tyme of her sicknes',[124] the majority of references which are specific relate to the cleaning of clothes, bedding and the house after the death. The reason for this is probably the obvious one: that, until death, cleaning of bedding and clothes was a function of attendance or nursing; after death it could not be described in this way. Lamentus Simms's cleaning and airing work was mentioned separately to her working as a nurse. If the types of cleaning referred to in these accounts are further broken down, it becomes apparent that there are many subsets. In addition to the cleaning of clothes and bedding in the time of the sickness, there is the *post mortem*

---

[120] On this subject see in particular Pelling, *Common lot*, 38–62.

[121] A possible example of such a payment is 'paid for spices and apothecarie wares for the deceased John Walter in the tyme of [his] sicknes 1s': PRC 2/3/174, dated 1584. Several Canterbury 'apothecaries' served apprenticeships with grocers, for example Walter Southwell, a licensed surgeon usually described in these accounts as an apothecary, served an apprenticeship with Christopher Bridge, grocer, to 1601. Joseph Colfe, Jr, was described as both an apothecary and a grocer in the records of Canterbury freemen. Similar crossovers between apothecaries and grocers/merchants are to be noted in the Exeter register of freemen. See *Exeter freemen*, in particular records relating to Thomas Flea as an apothecary and as a merchant 1599, 1608–9, 1619–20, 1626 etc.

[122] PRC 19/3/88. This is the last-dated explicit reference to spices. One 1664 account has the entry 'paid to Mary Harebeetle for candles sugar nutmeggs and other such like necessaries spent in the time of the said deceased sicknes': PRC 19/3/37.

[123] PRC 19/6/57.

[124] PRC 21/8/254.

cleaning of clothes spoiled in the illness,[125] the cleaning of the house,[126] the airing of a house and clothes of people infected with plague,[127] and the cleaning of items, usually clothes, so they might be sold.[128] The last group might include many ordinary possessions, especially in plague-stricken houses, as in 'for washing the said deceaseds nettes and roppes mencioned in the inventary afforesaid that they might be without Dainger apprized'.[129] Sometimes, however, there was no illness context to the cleaning at all, as in the case of James Hazard, who was lost at sea and yet whose account, dated 1691, has the entry: 'paid for washing up the deceaseds linnen upon his death and for sope and starch'.[130] The same account includes a payment for cleaning of his 'rusty cutlass', again clearly to maximise saleability, not the result of its being soiled in his sickness. In some cases men were paid for airing the house or cleaning,[131] and in one case for cleaning clothes within a plague-infected house.[132] This variation on the traditional gender roles emphatically places purification in plague cases into a different context from most housework, which was exclusively a female occupation. Clearly, to include all this within the conceptual framework of nursing would not be correct: much of it relates to household work. Those entries which place cleaning in an attendance context might well be interpreted as attempts to keep the body clean through frequent changing of clothes and bedding in the sickness of the dying person, and these undeniably reflect an aspect of nursing.[133] But it is difficult to know where the limit may be drawn. Even if

---

[125] 'Paid unto certen women which watched with the deceased & attended on hym in the tyme of his sicknes & for washing of sheets bedding & other things which he did ruyn & stayne in his sicknes 11/8': PRC 21/12/372, dated 1593; 'paid to two woomen for laying forth of the said deceased and for cleaning and washing of Certaine lynen which was fowled about the said deceased in the tyme of her sicknes': PRC 20/7/345, dated 1626; 'to Wyddow Crickman & Goodwife Prince for watching with the deceased ... and laying him forth and washing his lynnen since his death': PRC 2/29/68, dated 1628; 'to Alice Day and to Avice Stuings (?) of Marden for their paines in watching & attending on the said deceased ... & for washing up the fowle lynnen after her death': PRC 2/24/87.
[126] 'Paid for soape to wash the said Testatrixes linnen & a mop to wash her house after her interment': PRC 20/13/404, dated 1684; 'paid for washing up the deceaseds linnen and cleaneing the house and scouring the pewter': PRC 2/42/81.
[127] 'To certeyne washwomen for washing up the fowle lynnen after the death of the said deceased and for cleaning the howse': PRC 2/24/55, dated 1624; 'paid for sope and washing the said deceaseds linnen and for cleansing and ayring the said deceaseds house after his death': PRC 19/3/99.
[128] 'To 2 women to washe the linnen & napes before it could be solde 20d (and for sope for the same 12d)': PRC 21/4/101.
[129] PRC 2/27/71.
[130] PRC 19/5/2.
[131] For example 'paid to goodman Ramsberie for beeing in the howse of the said deceassed after his deathe to ayer and sweeten the gooddes and thinges there': PRC 2/9/491.
[132] 'Paid to Cornelius Erines for hott waters <for them> [the family shut in the house] and for washing of a Packe of garments which lay in the infected house': PRC 2/34/298.
[133] For the development of cleaning of the body through the cleaning of linen in France

it were possible to define which elements of cleaning were part of nursing and which were not, a systematic application could not be applied. The problem is exacerbated by the fact that most non-nursing attendants were the same women who did the cleaning both before and after death.[134] This might be interpreted as evidence that many attendants were little more than hired helps and washerwomen, an argument which would support a previous hypothesis with regard to the pre-1650 period; but equally it could be argued that women experienced in attending final sicknesses were no less capable of housework than inexperienced women. Nurses too, it should be added, often washed linen in the post-1660 period.[135] They also took part in cleaning houses after death, for example 'paid to another nurse for her dyett and for wood and ayring of the said deceaseds house after the distemper aforesaid'.[136]

The part of a nurse's role which lies entirely outside the scope of this study (i.e. attendance to the dying) is the laying out, or 'laying forth' of the body after death. Of all the functions which could be undertaken by women, this was the most gender-exclusive apart from washing linen and 'nursing', there being only five cases of men helping with the socking and laying forth of the deceased.[137] One account dated 1615 includes a payment 'unto the weomen that socke & layd forth the said deceased after his death, which for some

see G. Vigarello (trans. J. Birrell), *Concepts of cleanliness: changing attitudes in France since the Middle Ages*, Cambridge 1988. Note, however, that cleaning was not always possible or viable: 'paid unto him [Thomas webb] for a mattress whereon the said Thomas laye in his sicknesse and for a coverlett and two blanketts and for a feather bolster and pyllowe which were spoyled with corruption and suche as noe man afterwards would use 20s': PRC 21/8/82.

134 For example, 'Paide to Heles widow for wasshing of the clothes and for watching with her one night' is an example of washing: PRC 2/6/492; 'paid to the weomen which did watche with and attend on the said deceased in the time of the sicknes where of he died & for washing the linnen & cleaning the howse of the said deceased after his death': PRC 2/22/35.

135 For example, 'paid to a nurse who attended on the said deecased in his sicknesse whereof he dyed and for her dyett and for laying the deceased forth and washing the linen': PRC 2/41/27, dated 1685; and 'paid to a nurse who did watch and attend on the said deceased Johanna when she died and for cleaning and washing up things': PRC 1/17/80, dated 1715.

136 PRC 19/3/114, dated 1668. Other possible examples are: 'paid unto Lamentus Simms widow who was put in as a nurse to attend the said deceased a little before she died and for the time she remained there afterwards for the cleaning and airing of the goods': PRC 1/12/96, dated 1667; and 'paid unto the Nurses and others uppon cleaning of the house wherein the said deceased dyed, viewing the writeings, appriseing the goodes and other chardges thereabouts': PRC 19/3/76, a plague case, dated 1665.

137 'To goodman Long for watching with him in his sicknes & socking him after his death iijs, and to goodwife Paul for the like, the like sum': PRC 2/24/70, dated 1622; 'to a man for watching with the said testator two nights in the time of his sickness and for laying him forth': PRC 2/30/52, dated 1630; 'to men which laid forth the said deceased as alsoe to the weomen which attended and watched with him in the tyme of his sicknes': PRC 20/8/482, dated 1627. Two cases of a man and a woman jointly laying forth the deceased are 'to Thomas Smythe of Wittersham aforesaid and his wife for laying forth and

reasons they were unwillinge and hardlie interested to doe although they had for their paines a verye large allowance viz' the summe of 10s' (the normal payment was 2s. throughout the seventeenth century).[138] Given the expectation that the nastiest body-cleaning tasks would be performed by women, it is unlikely that the five cases reflect a trend for men to deal with the most revolting situations: other special factors were probably the reason. Where men were concerned in attendance it was more usual for them only to attend or watch with the deceased until death, at which point women took over to lay forth and sock the corpse. As shown in tables 57 and 58, it was not unknown for the women performing this function to be described as nurses. Laying out was still done by nurses in nineteenth-century hospitals.[139] Thus the twenty-seven instances of nurses in East Kent laying forth the corpse should not be taken as an indication of their casual labour. Also it should be borne in mind that laying forth was only one of several funeral-related services that East Kent nurses might undertake. They might attend at the funeral,[140] or go around the houses to invite guests to the funeral.[141] Indeed the role of women helping at the funeral was important, as shown by many entries throughout the whole period which mention such assistance. The expectation that female deathbed attendants would serve food and wine at a funeral suggests a ritual or social role more complicated than that of simple availability.[142]

Household and family help

The accounts do not mention, of course, the nursing services provided freely by family and other household members. However, they do give some shadowy references to the huge quantity of unpaid care undertaken by next of kin and the household. One account has the intriguing entry, 'paid to two women for

socking the said deceaseds dead corpse': PRC 20/9/217, dated 1631; and 'paid to Thomas Alburne & widow Dun for laying the said deceased forth': PRC 2/40/24.
[138] PRC 20/3/214. With regard to usual payments, the following examples show considerable consistency, suggesting traditional or standard charges of about 2s. per body: socking & laying forth 2s.: PRC 2/30/31, dated 1629; socking and laying forth 3s.: PRC 2/32/21, dated 1633; socking and laying forth 2s.: PRC 2/33/21, dated 1636; socking and laying forth 8d.: PRC 2/34/153, dated 1638; laying forth 2s.: PRC 2/37/121, dated 1678; laying forth 2s.: PRC 2/39/117, dated 1680; laying forth 2s.: PRC 2/40/30, dated 1682: laying forth of two corpses by two women 4s.: PRC 2/40/185, dated 1684; laying forth of a corpse by two women and wrapping it in wool 3s.: PRC 2/40/225, dated 1684; laying forth 1s. 4d.: PRC 2/40/262, dated 1684; laying forth 2s.: PRC 2/41/53, dated 1686; laying forth 2s.: PRC 2/41/60, dated 1686; laying forth 2s.: PRC 2/42/28, dated 1692.
[139] Pelling, Common lot, 196.
[140] 'Paid to Ann Ralph a nurse who laid the deceased forth and for her attendance att the funerall': PRC 19/6/2, dated 1702.
[141] 'To the nurse for inviteing the guests': PRC 19/6/12, dated 1703.
[142] PRC 20/13/216, dated 1681.

their helpe attendance and watching with the said deceased in the time of his sicknes at such times as the said murtons familie could not performe the office'.[143] It sounds as if the paid helpers were a stand-in for a preferred – and thus probably known – family of helpers, Murton being a basket-maker of Faversham noted elsewhere in the document. Another account includes a payment for 'a pound of candles to watche with the deceased' in his sickness, and a payment for socking the body, but no payment for the watching itself, which may well have been undertaken by members of the family.[144] Given the wide array of household work which attendants undertook, it is relevant to point to those provisioning and keeping payments where the deceased's widow was the payer, for example 'paid unto the said deceaseds widdow for money expended by her in the time of the said deceaseds sicknes, for necessaryes for housekeeping ... 38s'.[145] While it is true that such a payment is ostensibly just for housekeeping, 'necessaryes' could include many items purchased with a remedial or other health-related purpose, and many payments to attendants for 'keeping' were in effect little or nothing more than reimbursements for provisions and the effort of obtaining them.

The few accounts in which household attendance is regularly mentioned are those cases where a person died in another person's house. When this happened it was permissible to claim reimbursements paid to the host, his family and servants. Hence there are several dozen references to payments for servants, such as 'paid to Richard Reynolds for the helpe of his servantes attendynge the said Frances Lychepoole in the tyme of this sicknes 2s',[146] or 'giuen to the maydes of the howse where the said deceased died for their paynes and care towards him in his sicknes wherof hee died 4s'.[147] These payments, usually to maidservants in the house where the person died, use much the same language as the payments to attendants who were specifically brought in to attend the dying person. Some stress 'attending',[148] others stress 'pains-taking',[149] and others 'watching'.[150] Some include attendance at the

---

[143] PRC 2/34/156.
[144] PRC 21/15/125.
[145] PRC 20/12/59.
[146] PRC 2/4/359.
[147] PRC 20/7/186.
[148] For example, 'paide to a maide servante of the howse wherein the saide testator laye sicke for attending on him in the tyme of his sicknes wherof hee dyed 1s 8d': PRC 2/13/356, dated 1603; 'to a maide servaunt for attendinge the saide deceased in the tyme of his sicknes whereof he dyed': PRC 2/20/255.
[149] For example, 'paid to the payde servantes of Mr Valentine Everard for theire paynes taken with the said deceased in the tyme of his sicknes': PRC 2/17/250; 'bestowed on the servants at the red lion for their paynes taken with the said deceased whilest hee lay sicke there': PRC 2/33/12.
[150] For example, 'giuen unto the maydservant of the sayd Richard Peen for her paynes in attending on and watching with the said deceased in the tyme of the sicknes whereof he dyed': PRC 20/5/184; 'paid to Mr Bretts servant for watching with the said deceased in his sicknes and attendance at the funeral': PRC 20/13/163.

burial,[151] and others provisioning in the form of firewood or candles during the sickness.[152] Thus the full range of services associated with paid nursing help are also to be found in contexts of servants acting as helpers, which normally would not merit any payment other than their regular wages. There is even a case of a man acting as a helper,[153] and every so often the wife of the host.[154] The majority of servants in other people's houses were paid low wages, more in keeping with gratuities, and normally not exceeding 3s. This might set them apart from paid attendants, but equally it might reflect a short period of illness, for a long period would probably have resulted in the sick man being removed to his own home. In some cases servants attended and other women were brought in to 'watch' with the patient.[155] Those payments to servants which are of high value tend to be cases where a servant of the deceased was paid wages along with a payment for attendance.[156] That a servant of the deceased might perform the full range of attendance, washing and deathbed assistance is made clear in the payment 'to Margaret Grantham the said deceaseds {maid} <woman> servant for wages due and owing to her by the said deceased at the time of his death and for her attendance of the said deceased in the time of his sickness whereof he died and at his death and for washing of the said deceaseds linnen after his death 40s'.[157] Here the attendance clearly has the character of household work, a model strongly supported in two further payments to servants: 'paid to two servant maydes which attended upon the said deceased and his wife and children at the time of theire sicknesse the one being hired and tooke in of purpose for that time and the other being a servant mayd before 70s'.[158] Finally, there is the only reference in which a servant is directly referred to as a 'nurse': 'paid to the

---

[151] For example, 'to the maids of the howse for their paines taken with the deceased in his said in his sicknes (sic) and for helping at the buriall': PRC 2/24/24; 'paid to Mrs Pulley the vicars wife of Throwley in whose house the deceased died for her and her servantes paynes taken with the said deceased in the time of her last sickness and for use of the house and their helpe till after her Burialls': PRC 2/34/127.

[152] 'Paid more unto the said Stephen Lacy for his maids attendance uppon the said deceased in the time of the sickness whereof he died and for beere and fireing spent at the same tyme 20s': PRC 19/3/100.

[153] 'Paid to the said Widow Mantle for a mans service and help for the space of tenn or twelve weekes in the said deceased testator his roome whilest hee languished of the sicknes and indisposition of body whereof he died': PRC 2/34/45.

[154] 'Paid to the wife of John Bromdred of Wye in whose house the deceased testator died for attending him the testator in the time of his sickness whereof he died and for dyet and necessaries for him in the time of his sicknes': PRC 2/28/45.

[155] PRC 2/13/356. This account includes several such entries, for example 'paid to certeine women for watching with the saide Testator by the space of eleven dayes and nightes in the tyme of his sicknes ... 4s 8d'.

[156] For example, 'paid to John Fowlie of Ashford servant of the said deceased due to him by the said deceased for his wages & for attending of the familie of the said deceased in the tyme of their sicknes 26s 8d': PRC 2/16/32.

[157] PRC 20/9/269.

[158] PRC 19/1/22, a plague case.

Widdow Claringbole formerly the deceaseds servant and Nurse at his death for debt to her due by the said deceased 49s 2d'.[159] Thus, from an examination of household and family help in these accounts, there seems to be every indication that it reflects the nature and range of the attendance purchased on behalf of the dying in the wider parish community, with the obvious condition that the limit of sick-nursing expertise (as opposed to household work) was that of the most experienced woman in the household. Excluding this condition, household help seems to have largely followed the model of household work: provided by family members freely, or by servants in return for wages, and mostly with little or no specialised knowledge. That it was separately conceived from the paid attendance of more experienced women available in the latter part of the seventeenth century is suggested by there being only one reference to a servant acting as a 'nurse', and this to a widow, presumably a woman with some experience of nursing the dying.

Other counties

Those Wiltshire, Berkshire and West Sussex accounts which were correctly indexed contain twenty-two references to 'nursing'.[160] Twelve of these predate the Interregnum, and all but one of these is undoubtedly for wet-nursing or nursing children. The exception is an entry in a 1613 account which reads: 'Imprimis to the nurse for her wages'.[161] After the Restoration, one of the ten payments was for nursing a child; the other nine were for nurses' attendance or simply 'paid for nurses'. A 1675 Salisbury account distinguishes between nurses and watchers: 'paid to the Nurses & watchers for attendance in the sicknesse of the deceased'.[162] Only two payments give specific lengths of time of nurses' service: a 1693 Wiltshire account records payment of eight weeks' 'wages' to the nurses (2s. 6d. per week) and a 1708 Berkshire account, in which the patient suffered from smallpox, records a payment 'to two Nurses for Three Weeks attendance each vpon the deceased in his Sickness of the small pox at 15s. per week, 90s.'.[163] The high payment in respect of smallpox is particularly interesting as it is almost equivalent to the highest payments found in East Kent for nursing smallpox cases.

Turning to other nursing-related words, a number of close comparisons with East Kent are apparent. 'Keeping' was defunct as a service descriptor by the time of the Interregnum, the last such references being dated 1639

---

159 PRC 20/12/207.
160 For the problems with regard to the indexing of nursing entries in these counties see Mortimer, 'Medical assistance', i. 131–2.
161 WSRO, EpI/33/1613/16. The nurse in question was described as a servant earlier in the account.
162 WRO, P4/1674/13.
163 WRO, P2/B/1155; BRO, D/A1/198/38B (Berkshire accounts, 255).

(Wiltshire) and 1631 (Berkshire). No 'poor' person is noted as attending or watching after 1624 in Berkshire or 1631 in Wiltshire.[164]'Attendance' was by far the most commonly used term, appearing in approximately two-thirds of instances, with a regular disbursement throughout the period available for study (1590–1690). 'Watching', normally paid at a day-and-night rate rather than a weekly rate, merited payments of 4d. per day in West Sussex in 1611, 1614, 1617 and 1684, the same rate as in Kent.[165] Watching and attendance in Berkshire and West Sussex were undertaken by teams of helpers, as shown in entries such as 'for 3 women for watching with the deceased in the time of his sicknes',[166] or, explicitly, in the 1617 account of Thomas Meolls:[167]

Paid unto Joan Mather for attending the said deceased in his sickness one whole week, day and night, being unpaid at the time of his decease	3s. 6d.
Item paid unto Bridget Harrison for the like attendance 3 days and 2 nights, being unpaid at his death	2s.
Item paid her <husband> for three nights watchinge with the deceased being unpaid as abovesaid	1s.
Item paid William Hamkin for one nightes watchinge with the said deceased as aforesaid	4d.
Item paid unto Goodwife Beery for wasshinge the deceaseds lynnen and for watchinge him in his sicknes, unpaid as aforesaid	2s.
Item to John Staker for watchinge one nighte unpaid as aforesaid	4d.
Item paid unto Agnes Burry her 2 nightes watchinge	8d.

With regard to male assistance, as the above account reveals men were also paid as watchers in West Sussex; they were also sometimes paid as 'attendants',[168] and in one instance the same sort of justification is given for employing men in West Sussex as in East Kent: 'paid unto three men which watched with the said Tobie Hull by the space of one weeke in the time of his sicknes duringe which tyme he was very unrulie & had to be governed 16s.'.[169] Very occasionally, a man might be paid for laying out the corpse, for example 'paid {a Man} <Philipp Tayler> to lay out the Corps 6d'.[170] And occasionally, as in East Kent, payment might be made to attendants in kind, such as 'allowed to [blank] Gybbs in part of payment for his paynes in keeping of the said John and Alice and their famylie in the sicknes tyme, and

---

[164] BRO, D/A1/182/44A; WRO, P3/C/165.
[165] WSRO, EpIV/10/1/11, EpI/33/1613/3, EpI/33/1617/2, EpI/33/1684/42.
[166] BRO, D/A1/212/163E, dated 1593.
[167] WSRO, EpI/33/1617/2.
[168] Other examples are WSRO, EpI/33/1600/1, dated 1600; EpI/33/1684/42, dated 1684.
[169] WSRO, EpI/33/1617/6, dated 1617.
[170] This took place in respect of a Wiltshire man whose account was dated 1677: WRO, D1/41/3/20/127.

the trymmyng of the house till Michaelmas aforesaide, viz ii kyttells 2s. 6d., 2 pewter dishes 12d., one bushell of wheate 2s. 6d., one bushell and a half of barley 2s.'.[171] Names have been left blank in this entry for later insertion, suggesting that the accountant did not know the attendants well enough to be sure of them. Finally a last point of comparison is the variation in the levels of remuneration. In Kent it was noted that attendance could vary from 1s. 6d. when the patient was relatively poor to 8s. or more when the patient was suffering from a contagious illness. In Berkshire, Wiltshire and West Sussex, four days nursing (broadly defined) could range from as low as 2s. 6d. (as in Wiltshire in 1693) to as much as 8s. (as in West Sussex in 1598).[172] Other examples are the 3s. 6d. per week paid to Joan Mather in 1617 (West Sussex), and 4s. per week to 'Margaret May for 10 weeks attendance upon her in her sicknesse' in Berkshire in 1664.[173]

Bearing in mind such evidence, and also the paucity of these 300 references for three counties compared to nearly 2,500 for East Kent,[174] it may tentatively be said that the East Kent experience was largely borne out across central southern England. There are only two noted differences: the terms 'nurse' and 'nursing', which had become popular and widely used in East Kent by 1690, were only very rarely used in central southern England at this time. This could be a result of the limited number of accounts and the way in which they were indexed; but it could be expected that references to 'nurses' would have been picked up in the indexing process as 'medical' or 'illness'-related at least as often as 'keeping in the time of his sickness'. The other major difference is that only one account specifies a 'contractual rate' for nursing: all other rates are deduced from the periods of time specified. The one specific reference to a rate appears in the late (1708) account for a bargemaster of Abingdon mentioned above: two women nursing a smallpox case at 15s. each per week (the highest level of nursing remuneration of any sort in any of the accounts examined).[175] If the contractual system of 'attendance' and 'nursing' noted in respect of so many East Kent accounts was common across central southern England in the seventeenth century, at least a few more references might have been expected.

Nursing, like medicine, reached a watershed in the two decades 1640–60. Until then the term 'nursing' was rarely applied to sick-nursing in provincial southern England. The wider parish community might be involved in attending and watching, including men but with an emphasis on employing poor women on account of their cheapness, for long periods. The models of

---

171 WSRO, EpI/33/1583/1, dated 1583.
172 WRO, P2/B/1155; WSRO, EpI/33/1598/11.
173 BRO, D/A1/214/109C.
174 These figures exclude references expressly for provisioning and boarding when it is not clear who was buying the food or where the deceased was boarded.
175 *Berkshire probate accounts*, 255.

service may be likened to a household servant's remit of washing clothes and bedding, cleaning the room, making a fire in the patient's chamber if necessary, fetching food and feeding the patient. One other non-servant role may be added to this list: that of watching with the dying by night. Apart from instances of plague and smallpox, which may have involved familiarity with the illness and the risks of attendance, there is no strong evidence that the men, poor women, maids and boys who were paid to attend upon and watch with the dying in the late sixteenth and early seventeenth centuries had any more than the average level of medical knowledge.

The implications of this argument for women providing paid medical help in serious illnesses are obvious. Generally speaking, nursing functions did not include a significant medical element. Those few women who were sought out from afar for their medical skills stand in great contrast to local helpers. But even these medically proficient women were often paid for skin-related or child-related knowledge, not general medical skills. This low volume of paid female medical care on behalf of the dying was mirrored, at least before 1650, in the majority of female sick-nursing services being subsumed within household work, except with regard to plague and smallpox nursing. That said, there was throughout the period a small body of medically-informed attendants and nurses who, in the event of an emergency, might themselves take a medical initiative on behalf of their patient. It is unlikely that this amounted to more than 10 per cent of all attendants in the period prior to 1640.

By 1660 the system of general attendance, by which all and sundry in a locality might be employed, regardless of age, gender and specialist knowledge, had clearly been replaced by a more formal approach to nursing. Experienced women almost exclusively came to dominate nursing roles, and were increasingly given the epithet or pretitle 'nurse' as an occupational identity in relation to sick care, not just wet-nursing and child care. The rise of nursing as an occupation is to be seen not only in the frequency with which the term came to be used but in language which specifically excluded some women from being termed nurses, as in 'for Doctors Nurses and other attendance the deceased Dying of the small pox'.[176] The implications of this change in the language is that, in addition to the 'household work' model of attendance, there was in this period a 'nursing' model. This seems to have required greater experience, and a degree of skill (to judge from Fuller's requirements), and it carried with it its own identity which made redundant old identities such as 'poor woman'. This was a form of attendance in which men, maids and boys did not participate, and for which rewards could sometimes be high. The very fact that a shift towards such exclusivity was accompanied not by a fall in nursing care but by a slight rise may be evidence that some of these more experienced women were concentrating on nursing as an occupation.

[176] PRC 2/36/6.

Unlike the earlier period, very few nurses acted independently of medical practitioners. They might not have been formally trained, or even full-time, and they were still a loosely organised group of widows and married women, but their part-time occupation had acquired a greater degree of respectability (having shed its connotations of poor labour), and was widely recognised as such across Kent in the late seventeenth century, and in other southern counties at the same time or not much later.

6

Plague and Smallpox

'for watching at the doores of the said deceaseds house to notifye the disease with Intent by God's blessing to preserve others from the infection'.[1]

It is both a truism and a regrettable limitation that very few specific diseases are mentioned in these accounts, and so it remains inevitable that what is charted in this book is an increasingly medicalised response to illness in general, with no sensitivity to which specific diseases or ailments were perceived to be treatable, and thus to which medical and social issues were perhaps driving change. However, it is possible to distinguish certain types of medical condition. In particular, plague and smallpox are often specified as the cause of death, or the reason why extensive and expensive nursing care was purchased. This chapter will therefore seek to answer a specific question: is there any evidence that medical responses to plague and smallpox were different from those to other sicknessess?

The key problem is lack of knowledge: there is simply no information on how many people suffered from either of these illnesses. Although it is possible to say that 10 per cent of all Status B males in East Kent are recorded as paying for medical assistance in the period 1600–19, it is impossible to establish how many of those suffered from plague. It would be possible to say how many accounts which mention plague also include medical or nursing assistance, but since the main reason for mentioning plague is to justify medical or nursing expenditure, this would not be a valid way of measuring the comparative use of external assistance in respect of plague. The costs of nursing and attending plague and smallpox cases could be very significant, approximately double the costs of nursing other ailments, but whether these services were as regularly purchased it is not possible to say. All that can be done is to investigate the nature of the response to these sicknesses, and to look for discrepancies.

If specific references to smallpox and plague are pooled with other descriptions of infectious illnesses, namely those described as the 'infection', 'visitation' and 'pestilence', and combined with cases in which more than one person was buried from a household, statistics for medical and nursing strategies in infectious cases may be compared with those for which there is no definite infectious context.

The most significant differences between tables 65 and 66 relate to

---

[1] PRC 2/33/34.

Table 65
Type of assistance in contagious diseases

Date	Total medical and nursing	Medical only	Nursing only
1570–1599	76	9%	75%
1600–29	105	9%	65%
1630–49	73	15%	48%
1660–89	100	9%	51%
1690–1719	35	26%	9%

Note: 'Contagious' here refers to all accounts with medical or nursing assistance in which smallpox or plague is mentioned, or more than one member of the household died. The percentages are the proportion of all those for whom there was some medical or nursing expenditure.

Table 66
Type of assistance in non-contagious diseases

Date	Total medical and nursing	Medical only	Nursing only
1570–99	349	14%	70%
1600–29	805	23%	58%
1630–49	500	36%	58%
1660–89	999	58%	14%
1690–1719	264	59%	9%

payments for nursing, and medical help in isolation from nursing. After 1660 more than half of all interventions in 'non-contagious' cases were due to medical practitioners alone, and paid nursing was not required. But where 'contagious' illnesses were noted in the period 1660–1719, almost all the dying were attended by helpers, attendants and nurses, and just 14 per cent received medical care without nursing aid. Thus nursing seems to have been of considerably greater significance in these cases of dreaded, infectious or contagious diseases than in other cases.

If the table of contagious cases is broken down into its constituent elements (*see* tables 67 and 68), the contrast between contagious and uncertain illnesses is even more pronounced. Of those contagious cases which received some external help, between eight- and nine-tenths was provided by nurses or attendants, not medical practitioners. For those households with plague, nursing was considerably more frequently recorded than medical intervention; and, until the post-1690 period, this may also be said for smallpox. It is tempting to say that most households could not provide the nursing for plague and smallpox cases as they could for other fatal diseases.

Such figures support the hypothesis that the level of nursing of or attendance upon victims of plague or smallpox was subject to different influences

Table 67
Nature of assistance purchased on behalf of plague victims

Date	Total medical and nursing	Medical only	Nursing only
1570–99	19	16%	68%
1600–29	35	11%	46%
1630–49	27	7%	37%
1660–89	32	0	66%

Table 68
Nature of assistance purchased on behalf of smallpox victims

Date	Total medical and nursing	Medical only	Nursing only
1570–99	1	0	100%
1600–29	7	0	71%
1630–49	19	11%	79%
1660–89	28	4%	61%
1690–1719	11	9%	18%

when compared with other afflictions. With regard to plague in particular, even in the last decade of the disease's prevalence, two-thirds of sufferers paid for nursing help alone, whereas most diseases by this time provoked more medical reactions. This hints at another important difference between illnesses generally and these horror illnesses: in most cases of plague, the physician or surgeon did not attend the dying man and his family. The diet drinks and physic which were purchased were obtained by the nurses and attendants, or an intermediary (even the local pest master in a few cases) and administered as part of the attendants' task.

This brings back into focus the question of the extent to which nurses took the medical initiative. As was made clear in chapter 5, in the absence of attendance by medical practitioners, nurses sought and administered medicine in perhaps 10 per cent of the cases they attended. If medical practitioners were reluctant to become involved in plague cases, they may have left the family and their nurses no option but to take a medical – or at least a medicinal – initiative themselves, if they deemed such an initiative desirable. Since early seventeenth-century medicalisation had encouraged people generally to think of health strategies in medicinal terms, there is every likelihood that many victims did seek medicinal solutions independently of a practitioner. So it is a moot point whether medical practitioners did or did not intervene personally and directly in plague and smallpox cases, or whether in their absence those directing the care strategy took the medical initiative themselves.

Wisdom to date, and the evidence so far presented, suggests that physi-

Table 69
Payments in cases of plague in East Kent

	1570–1649	1660–79
Apothecary	3	1
Doctor	2	4
Nurses	4	24
Helpers paid for attendance, keeping and watching	86	11
Surgeon	9	1
Uncertain, paid for physic or medicines	25	4
Pestmaster paid for medicine	5	0
Physician	4	0

Note: Figures do not include any ambiguous cases, such as 'pestilence', 'visitation' or suchlike.

cians shunned plague victims. Simon Forman was proud to be able to state that he did not leave London, like most physicians, during an outbreak, thereby suggesting that he was unusual. Even Richard Napier, who did treat plague victims himself when they came to him, refused personally to visit patients whom he knew to be infected.[2] Treatment of this affliction was more frequently nursing-assisted than medical practitioner-assisted. This fact is demonstrated even more emphatically in the graphic demonstration of individual payments to practitioners and nurses (broadly defined) in table 69. Although 'physicians' and 'doctors' were taking on the majority of medical cases after 1660, they hardly feature. Both before and after the Interregnum, members of the tripartite medical system were irregular participants in the care of victims of the plague: the 'regulars' were the attendants (before 1650) and nurses (after 1650). The nearest to 'regular' medical practitioners involved in the process were those men of uncertain occupation who supplied physic to the dying and their carers.

If nurses were the 'regulars' in infected houses, and taking a role in directing the care, what were they doing? They were, of course, performing much the same tasks that they might perform in other, non-infected houses: watching in the night, attending, keeping, cleaning and helping. But whether their medical role was significantly more substantial than the medical role of nurses in general is a different question.

The figures presented in tables 69 and 70 are based upon just 161 households with plague.[3] Nevertheless they consistently indicate a major differ-

[2] B. H. Traister, The notorious astrological physician of London: works and days of Simon Forman, Chicago 2001, 45; Sawyer, 'Patients, healers', 427, 435.
[3] For an explanation of why the figures in table 70 are ranges see Mortimer, 'Medical assistance', i. 308; ii. 157.

Table 70
Direction of medical strategies in plague cases in East Kent

	1570–1609 %	1610–49 %	1660–89 %	1690–1719 %
Accounts which record medical practitioners whose first-hand advice was or may have been given (practitioner-directed strategies)	16–32	20–51	22–63	25–31
Accounts which record nursing assistance but no medical practitioners or medical advice (home- or nursing-directed strategies)	68–79	49–71	37–74	69–75
Accounts which record only purchases of medicines and no medical advice nor nursing care (home-directed strategies)	0–5	0–9	0–4	0

ence from those recorded in table 63. There does not seem to have been a collapse in the proportion of cases in the 1630s–40s and the 1660s–1670s which were attended exclusively by nurses. With this in mind, the wording of the accounts is significant. Although the evidence is rarely explicit, it seems that nurses might administer – if not prescribe – diet drinks, purges and vomits. The following entry appears in an account devoid of other medical references:

> for the charge of a Nurse that attended Stephen Mockett one of the said deceaseds children who was likewise shutt upp and visited with the said distemper [the 'pestilence'] and for a purge and a vomitt, sugar, strong waters and other materials spent in the time of their visitation.[4]

Equally ambiguous, in that it does not explicitly state that the payee administered the physic himself, although it points very strongly in that direction, is the following entry:

> Item to David Maryland or his assignes for keeping of & attendance vppon the aforesaid Elizabeth Cooper deceased and her three children in the time of her sicknes whereof shee and twoe of them dyed the said sicknes beeing an infection of the plague for watching with Phisicke victualls and other necessaries for the said deceased and her children and such as attended on them all the time which this accomptant paid by order and appoyntment of the maior of the cittie of Canterburye.[5]

There is no mystery as to why few medical practitioners attended plague houses with less frequency than other diseases. As Paul Slack has pointed

4 PRC 19/4/25, dated 1668.
5 PRC 2/17/292, dated 1613.

out, many simply fled.[6] Sawyer has suggested that the practice of locking up the occupants of a plague-infected house served to keep practitioners out.[7] Although the intention of isolation was to keep infected people inside the house rather than non-infected people out, a description of a house shut up in this way provides further evidence for nurses apparently acting independently of practitioners. The account is that of one John Chasmer, whose house

> was imediately before & after his death visited with the plague or other like contagious sicknes whereof divers several persons dyed out of the said house within short time one of another, as namely first a child of his owne, then one of his daughters beeinge children which he kept, afterward himselfe & his wife, & shortly after one [Burch?] a woman that attended the sick people of the house By reason of which visitacion the same house was shutt up from about the 20th of October last past until about the latter end of January next following, the charge of provision for the said house during which time, both in meate & drinke, in phisicke & medicines, in nurces & tenders, in warders and searchers and such like, as alsoe of the burial of the said John Chasmer & his wife & such others of the house as died.[8]

It is noticeable in this case that, although there was a payment for 'physicke & medicines' there was no reference to a medical practitioner, just 'nurces and tenders'. It may be that one was subsumed within 'physic' but it seems more likely that herein there is a model for medical help in the time of the plague: the purchasing of medicines which were then either self-administered or administered by an attendant. Logically, unless the advice as to what should be taken was left to the apothecary, then it was the nurses and family who selected the medical option and directed the medical aspects of the care programme as well as the palliative aspects.

However, some practitioners did attend plague cases (*see* table 70). The 1668 account of Thomas Figg includes a payment which reads 'unto two doctors for their fees in coming to visit the said deceased (he dying of the distemper commonly called the plague) and for physick by them administered to him and the rest of the family, in all £4 5s'.[9] Similarly, the 1638 account of John Barrowe specifies a payment to

> Mr Israel Vanderslaert of Ashford phisitian and others for phisick and Chirurgicall thinges applied to the said deceased and administred in his life tyme and also to all or most part of his familie for a long tyme after his decease, the better (by God's blessing) to preserve them from the Contagious fever aforesaid, and for often visiting them in the tyme they were shutt upp or kept in as aforesaid £10.[10]

6   Slack, *Impact of plague*, 32.
7   Sawyer, 'Patients, healers', 427.
8   PRC 20/10/202, dated 1638.
9   PRC 1/13/38.
10 PRC 20/10/43. This 'fever' is elsewhere described as plague.

Several of the most widely-used physicians are named unambiguously as attending plague cases. Two further payments which may be singled out in this context are those to 'Mr Charles Annot of Canterburie chirurgion for medycine for the famylie of the said deceassed visited and infected as afore is saide with the plawge and for his paines and diligence in attending on the said famylie divers weekes together verie carefully £8 13s 4d', and 'paid to one Mr Dade a physician of Sittingbourne for physick ministered by him to the said James Drewry in his last sickness whereof he died and for visitation of him in the time ... £1'. It has to be said that the victims of plague who received the personal attentions of named physicians were rich (John Barrowe had a estate of £2,138; the patients seen by Charles Annot and John Dade had estates of £732 and £436 respectively). Excluding the role of the Sandwich pest master, there are only five cases of Status C and D individuals affected by plague being attended by males who may or may not have been medical practitioners.[11] Richard Napier's reluctance to visit or receive plague victims seems to have been representative of the East Kent practitioners too.

On the strength of this the model of care for plague victims may be clarified. Few medical practitioners attended plague cases, and when they did it was generally only when the victim was wealthy. Surgeons might treat plague sores, but usually only after the danger of infection had passed: most references to surgeons in this capacity are in the context of healing the sores still carried by children of the deceased after they had recovered from the disease. Most of the attendance was performed by attendants and nurses for high fees, with an acknowledgement of risk, and normally on the basis of a weekly rate, implying a form of verbal contract. There are no instances at all of payments for occasional 'watching', paid on a daily or nightly rate. Attendants – always women after 1640 – performed functions along the lines of the housework model established in chapter 5 but might supplement their care of the dying with purges, vomits and diet drinks purchased from doctors and apothecaries.[12] In some plague cases nurses may have taken over the responsibility for

---

[11] These are 'paide by this accomptant vnto a surgeon for attending with the twoe children of the saide deceassed after their father (sic) deathe by the space of ix weekes at 11s the weeke the saide twoe children beeing then sicke of the plague, & the surgeon abideing all that tyme in howse with them': PRC 2/9/55, dated 1596; 'paid to Mr Christopher Waters of Ashford aforesaid phisitian for more phisicke and other necessaries applied by him to the said deceased': PRC 2/27/158, dated 1626; 'paid vnto Francis Taverner of sandwich aforesaid for helpe and attendance of the said deceased and the rest that were visited in his family they beeing shutt upp {nine monthes} ten weekes at 8s the week': PRC 2/34/275, dated 1639; 'paid to Mr Wright of Maidstone for physick by him administred unto the said deceased his wife and children, and also for other necessary things fetched from the Apothecaryes <shopp> in the time of their being shutt upp and visited': PRC 19/3/124, dated 1667; and 'paid to Mr Trowts of feversham for Phisicke which he administred to the said deceased': PRC 20/9/91, dated 1630.

[12] There are three references dated 1639 to men attending plague cases: PRC 19/1/87, PRC 2/34/275 and PRC 1/3/31. Of these the first is in conjunction with a woman and

directing the care from the next of kin, and sought and administered medicines themselves, rather than turning to medical practitioners. Thus it might
be said that, in some cases, nurses acted as 'plague-physicians', directing the
care for the dying person, seeking and fetching medicines from physicians
and apothecaries, and administering these medicines to the patient.

The other aspect of plague which must be mentioned is that of public
health. By the late sixteenth century plague had very well-recognised public
health implications, and these are reflected in the Order in Council of 1578,
by the terms of which constables had the duty of sealing up plague houses
for the duration of the visitation.[13] As a result plague was perhaps the only
disease which the sufferer and his family did not have sole authority to
combat. Warders were assigned to watch the house, and the occupants of
a plague house were charged for their attendance. Women and, occasionally, surgeons were paid to search the living or dead body to discover the
nature of illness in cases where plague was suspected.[14] Canterbury and the
larger towns had sworn 'searchers' whose duty was expressly to investigate
possible cases of plague.[15] Such appointments might be at the order of a
public authority, a JP, a mayor of a town or the constable of a parish. Attendants within the house could also be appointed by a public authority.[16] In
the case of urban plague there were pest houses where the plague-stricken
might be taken to recover or die. Thus, perhaps more than with any other
disease, plague victims could be locked into a system of care and management in which they were passive sufferers, unable to direct their own treatment strategy unless they were relatively wealthy.

Although this was no doubt true, the public system of care as revealed in
these accounts was an active one, at least with regard to the Sandwich area,

the other two could be payments to nondescript medical practitioners. Otherwise the
last payment to a man for attending a plague victim as a helper (paid for 'watching and
attending') was in 1614: PRC 20/3/101.

[13] *Berkshire probate accounts*, p. xv.

[14] A rare case of a surgeon being paid to search for the disease appears in a 1582 account:
'Paid by this accomptant to a surgion to go into the howse in the tyme of sicknes to take
knowledge of the disease that he was sicke of': PRC 2/2/39.

[15] 'Payd unto Gyles Clarke the sworne searcher of the Citty of Canterbury for searching
and viewing the severall bodyes of the said deceased parties before they could be admitted
to buryall 6s; [next entry] for the Beadle of Canterbury for … the same service 5s': PRC
19/3/76, dated 1665.

[16] For example 'Item paid to Widow Bing a Poore sercher and keeper of people infected
of the plague appointed by those in authoritie for three full weekes and about foure daies
keeping and attending the said deceased in the time of the said infeccion and of this
accomptant and his family after his death in the tyme of that then visitacion before they
were sett free (after the rate of 6s the weeke being the summe by authority appointed for
her' [25s. was paid]. The following entry reads 'Item paid to Marie Bennet another keeper
appointed by Mr Maior of Dovor for the like purpose and for the like tyme, a great parte
of which she did looke to the said Bing which was also infected whilest she was in the
said deceaseds house as a keeper or attendant aforesaid': PRC 2/34/251, dated 1637.

where the 'pest master' took a proactive role outside the pest house as well as within it.[17] One reference reads 'payd to the pestmaster of Sandwich for visiting the said Daniell in the time of his infectious sicknes wherof hee died and for drinkes given to the said Daniell in that time to prevent death if it might have beene'.[18] In addition, a number of references to the Sandwich pest master's 'attendance' and provision of diet drinks and medicines may be noted without any reference to the diseased family's being accommodated at the pest house.[19] One account is explicit in that it notes a payment to 'Peeter Boutam the Pest Master of Sandwich for phisick & drinkes and attendance of the said deceased and the rest of his family in the time of the visitation' and then mentions that the said deceased and his whole family were 'shut-up' for eight or nine weeks. The fact that the whole family was isolated suggests that they remained in their own house, and that the pest master visited them there.

The proactive role of the 'system of care' in plague cases also included non-medical elements: plague wardens – exclusively male – who ostensibly were paid to watch each infected house but who might also run errands and fetch food, fuel and medicines for those within. Indeed, the publicly-appointed warden was not so much the guard of an imprisoned household as their (extra-mural) servant. Instances of wardens being paid for external chores are not uncommon, and cover all the plague-affected decades of the seventeenth century. Two representative examples are:

> Item paid and laid out for provisions of dyett and all other necessaries spent and laid out upon all the parties in such time as they were kept shutt up for the sicknesses and for sundry <persons> to watch and ward at the doore of the deceased by the space of eight weekes together which was done by the command of his majesties Justice of the Peace to prevent others from coming thither to take the like infection and for diverse journies and other charges in that time expended.[20]

and

> Item paid unto John Wiber being imployed as a watchman to attend uppon the said visitted and Carry them all necessaries, for his constant attendance and service in that way by the space of eleven weekes, after the rate of 10s per week.[21]

---

[17] 'Payd for drinkes made in the tyme of his sickines att the pest master': PRC 2/16/172, dated 1612.

[18] PRC 2/34/297, dated 1638.

[19] For example, PRC 2/34/298, dated 1639; PRC 2/34/275, dated 1639; and PRC 2/27/172, dated 1626.

[20] PRC 19/1/22, dated 1641.

[21] PRC 19/3/76, dated 1665. Two other full entries are 'paide to Thomas Gosling of Mersham whoe was by the Justices of Peace appointed to attend the deceassedes howse whilest yt was infected with the plauge. for his travaile and paynes in doing the same

The high rate of pay for male watchers (as high as nursing rates for plague), suggests that there may have been a perception of some risk attached to the role of warden, similar to the role of attendant or nurse.

The unique public health aspect of plague makes it subject to very different choices and strategies. The family and sick person were not always able to decide for themselves on medical or nursing care, and sometimes not even able to decide where they might suffer the disease, if in town, for they might be removed to a pest house. They could not always choose those who attended them, and if they did secure the services of a nurse, sometimes from a more distant parish, they had to pay high wages. Therefore in many ways plague is not comparable with other diseases, even other infectious diseases. Was smallpox, the other disease commonly singled out for mention, also subject to its own culture of treatment and containment?

Table 71 displays a pattern similar to that of plague. Roughly three-quarters of payments were in respect of attendance or (later) nursing; the remainder were divided between a range of practitioner types (but more medical practitioners appear after 1660 than before). High wages were paid in respect of smallpox, and attendants on smallpox cases were drawn from further afield; these aspects compare with plague and were different from usual nursing patterns. Smallpox also compares to plague in that occasional watching, paid for on a daily or nightly rate, did not take place: all attendance, including 'watching', was long-term and probably contractual. But these similarities mask a number of differences between the two diseases. Indeed, they mask the fact that the period 1640–60 – the period when 'attendants' were more commonly becoming known as 'nurses' – saw something of a watershed in smallpox treatment.

Prior to the Interregnum, nursing attendance on smallpox cases was comparable in some respects with plague. Very little evidence of medical practitioner involvement has been found in the accounts for this period (and this is true for all the counties examined, not just Kent). Thus the care strategy seems almost exclusively to have been directed by the nurses or the family itself. At the same time, references have been found to sufferers being restrained from going abroad with the disease.[22] While restricting movement

and for thinges laide owte and provided by him dureing that time': PRC 2/13/137, dated 1605; and 'paid to Jefferie Marten of Ashford for warding the howse of the said deceased in the tyme that it was infected with the plage & for fetching of victualls for him & his howshold whylest there they were infected with the plage 2s 4d': PRC 2/16/32, dated 1612.

[22] Examples of families being restrained (not necessarily by public order) within their houses are 'for meate and drinke for the said attendants while they soe attended and afterwards before they were fit to go abroad by reason of the said infection of the small pocks': PRC 20/11/329, dated 1635; 'for the charges in keeping of three servants and one apprentice for the space of four months and for the expense upon those which attended them all that time being everyone of them visited with the small pox until they were fully recovered and might without danger go abroad among other company without fear

Table 71
Payments in cases of smallpox in East Kent

	1570–1649	1660–79
Apothecary	0	2
Doctor	1	8
Helpers paid for attendance, keeping and watching	33	16
Nurses	1	31
Physician	1	3
Surgeon	0	2
Uncertain, paid for physic or medicines	3	7

Note: Figures do not include any ambiguous cases, such as 'visitation' or suchlike.

is not the same as shutting up the house, the absence of practitioner involve‑
ment and attendance prior to 1650 suggests that this amounted to much the
same thing. A slightly later account (1667) refers to a house being shut-up
by a JP.[23] But public health with regard to smallpox differed substantially
from plague in that there was no smallpox hospital in Kent in the manner of
a pest house. The direction of the strategy to cope with the disease remained
a private matter: no wardens were appointed by external bodies and attend‑
ants only very rarely. Treatment usually took place in the patient's own
home, as with most diseases. It is arguable that this aspect of smallpox care
– the private nature of dealing with the disease – encouraged greater interac‑
tion between patient and practitioner. Such had, of course, been common
among the upper classes before this period,[24] but after the Interregnum it
appears that the average patient and his household increasingly sought treat‑
ment from practitioners as well as nurses. The disease quickly became the
subject of private medical interactions with doctors over and above the mere
purchasing of diet drinks and vomits from apothecaries.[25] In other words,

or shuning': PRC 1/2/16, dated 1639; and 'paid to one __Pearson of Wye for attendance
on and looking to the said deceased and his family together with the goods and estate
he left in and about his house for a long time together till his goods could be prised, the
said infection over (?) passed and his children recovered and at liberty to go abroad': PRC
1/7/15, dated 1643.
[23] For a description of a smallpox-infected house (but one possibly also infected with
plague) being closed see 'paid in like manner unto one Bennett Rye and a Nurse for their
attendance upon and looking unto the said deceased and her family in the time of their
being shut up, as visited with the sickness and small pox': PRC 1/11/113, dated 1667.
[24] See, for example, G. S. Thompson, Life in a noble household, London 1937, 33–5,
39–40, 317–22.
[25] There are five accounts which relate to smallpox victims which do not carry refer‑
ences to nursing or medicine; these are dated 1629, 1637, 1649, 1669 and 1676. They
may reflect sudden deaths or failure to record medical expenditure: PRC 2/30/123; PRC
20/10/470; PRC 1/8/59; PRC 1/13/140; and PR C2/37/2 respectively.

Table 72

Direction of medical strategies in smallpox cases in East Kent

	1570–1609 %	1610–49 %	1660–89 %	1690–1719 %
Accounts which record medical practitioners whose first-hand advice was or may have been given (practitioner-directed strategies)	0–28	0	32–9	73–82
Accounts which record nursing assistance but no medical practitioners or medical advice (home- or nursing-directed strategies)	72–100	79–100	61–8	18
Accounts which record only purchases of medicines and no medical advice nor nursing care (home-directed strategies)	0	0–10	0	0–10

smallpox was initially an affliction, like plague, attended almost exclusively by nurses, but increasingly came to be overseen by medical practitioners (like diseases in general) in the late seventeenth century.

Most late seventeenth-century smallpox cases show regular expenditure on both nursing and medicine. It is interesting that although smallpox merited high weekly wages, the totals paid were considerably less than in cases of plague. There is only one payment specifically for care undertaken in respect of smallpox of more than £5; a payment of £6 11s. to 'three Nurses that did attend the said deceased in his sicknes ... which was the small pox' in Sandhurst (Kent) in 1675.[26] The highest practitioner's bill in respect of smallpox was the £2 6s. 6d. paid 'to Mr Relfe of Cranbrook the deceased's physician for physick given to the deceased in the time of his sickness and for divers visits afforded him in that time'.[27] Medical assistance was thus relatively affordable. Certainly it had become more accessible to smallpox patients. From the date of the account recording Mr Relfe's visit (1662) onwards, physicians were increasingly mentioned as personally administering physic to smallpox patients, and occasionally as visiting them: trends directly comparable with those noted for physicians in general, as shown in chapter 3. The 1669 account of an East Sutton man records a payment 'unto Doctor

---

[26] PRC 2/36/196. Higher payments are either ambiguous as in the one payment of more than 100s. to a doctor which is described as a debt ('paid to Dr Sampson a debt [of 140s.] due and owing unto him by the deceased at his death': PRC 1/18/12, dated 1716), or payments for accommodation and board. There are about twenty payments for plague nursing totalling more than £5.

[27] PRC 1/9/30, dated 1662.

Hartnap of Smarden for physick by him administered unto the said deceased in the time of his sicknes … as also for sending a horse and a man four several times to fetch the said doctor'.[28] The 1712 account of a Brook man includes two payments, one 'to Mr Toke phisitian for his iournyes & medicines had of him by the aforesaid deceaseds in their sicknesses aforesaid as by his bill' and another 'to Mr Murrell surgeon for his advice and attendance on the before mentioned deceased in their sicknesses they died of'.[29] Both of these were smallpox cases.

To judge from the 135 payments in respect of smallpox in these accounts, the social and medical approach to the disease shifted fundamentally in the late seventeenth century. Before 1640 the approach appears to have been predominantly disease-dominated, as victims were expected to remain in their houses, mostly unattended by medical practitioners, until they died or recovered under the direction of attendants. By 1700 most cases received both medical and nursing help. There was still an awareness that the disease was contagious and needed isolation, but, unlike plague victims, sufferers were not shunned by medical practitioners. In some places nurses continued to treat smallpox victims too. When the Abingdon bargemaster, Daniel Hyde, fell ill with smallpox in the early eighteenth century, 1s. 6d. was paid for 'the rent of a Room in another place for the deceaseds family whilest he was sick of the small pox'.[30] Two nurses were paid for attending him for three weeks at a rate of 15s. per week, and, separately, the 'watchers' were paid 10s. A further payment of £1 3s. 6d. was made to the apothecary and, from the absence of references to a physician or surgeon, it seems likely that whatever medicines were purchased were administered by the nurses themselves (the family being kept elsewhere). Although physicians and surgeons did attend smallpox patients personally, nurses retained a medicine-administering role in respect of this disease which had been theirs by default prior to 1650 in cases of infectious fatal illnesses. It is no surprise to read Gideon Harvey's statement in 1683 that 'nurses effectively competed with physicians in the management of smallpox'.[31]

In conclusion, in answer to the question of whether there were distinct medical responses to plague and smallpox, the answer is most certainly yes. Plague in particular is not comparable with the generality of diseases, for it did not follow the observable pattern of medicalisation with regard to fatal conditions; this may be connected with some unique features, particularly the public nature of determining a disease strategy. Smallpox treatment, which was in many respects comparable with plague treatment until about 1660, began to resemble the general pattern of medicalisation much more closely after this date. In addition, there were significant differences in the

---

[28] PRC 1/14/22.
[29] PRC 19/6/59. Each of these practitioners was paid 30s.
[30] BRO, D/A1/198/38b, quoted in *Berkshire probate accounts*, 255.
[31] Pelling, *Common lot*, 199.

ways in which nurses and medical practitioners approached these diseases. It is clear that the nurses' help was practically the only assistance available to the average plague-stricken and pre-1650 smallpox-infected household. By default, then, tenders and nurses retained responsibility for directing the care of those dying of these diseases for much longer than they did with regard to other diseases, which showed signs of starting to be medicalised from the 1620s. With a growing expectation of medicinal applications from the 1620s, this meant that nurses attending plague and smallpox cases sometimes also acquired a medical role. In smallpox cases after 1660 medical practitioners were paid for advice, and it may be that they gained control of the disease strategy. But they were not always called in, and in such cases the medicalised role of the nurse was important. In East Kent, medical practitioners seem to have been only partially successful in bringing smallpox within their control. Of the forty-five cases noted in these accounts after 1660, fewer than half – probably only seventeen – were treated by medical practitioners; the care strategies of the remainder were directed by nurses or family members.[32] Of the thirty-nine cases of plague after 1660, doctors, physicians and surgeons were paid in respect of only eight. Highly-paid nurses were responsible for directing treatment in probably 70 per cent or more of the last two decades of plague cases, compared to 12–25 per cent of illnesses in general.

[32] For discussion of nursing as a medical approach to smallpox see ibid.

Conclusion

This study has sought to chart the changing relationships between the seriously ill and dying and their medical practitioners and nurses between 1570 and 1720. A summary of the major findings has to begin with the principal trend noted in the first two chapters: there was a dramatic and widespread increase in the proportion of dying people receiving medical help or purchasing physic in the last days and weeks of their lives in the seventeenth century. The increase in East Kent may be measured as varying from a minimum of +360 per cent for urban higher status groups (+550 per cent for their rural counterparts) to +1,130 per cent for rural lower status groups (+600 per cent for their urban counterparts), measured across thirty-year periods centred on c. 1585 and c. 1705 (see appendix). Similar increases in medicalisation, varying according to social status and geographic location, seem to have been experienced across all the four counties included in this study, excluding only lower-status patients in rural parts of Wiltshire. Given the probable under-recording of medical strategies in the accounts, there is little doubt that the majority of dying people (possibly excluding the destitute and very poor) in the last decades of the seventeenth century and the first two decades of the eighteenth obtained some form of occupationally defined medical treatment or advice. This is in distinct contrast with the situation a century earlier, at which time most paid interventions were exclusively those of an attendance or palliative nature.

There are many ways of interpreting this development. Given the opportunities presented by the source material, this study has concentrated largely on the economic and practical aspects of medical care. In particular, it has been demonstrated that, as medical responses to life-threatening situations increased in popularity, payments for nursing care did not increase significantly in number. Rather the nature of paid assistance during a fatal sickness shifted from being described in terms of constant palliative care to being described in terms of intermittent medical assistance, in the form of practitioners' occupations and payments for medicines.

This change raises the question of how it was possible for so many more people to be supplied with medicine and medical assistance at the end of the century than at the start. This is especially pertinent in view of there being just as many practitioners available in 1620–40 as in 1670–1710. It seems probable that the increased availability of medical services to the seriously ill was almost certainly dependent on the changing character of medical interventions. Particularly noteworthy are practitioners' increased propensity to serve clientele from rural areas, to dispense more medicines, to travel to patients in rural areas, to settle in greater numbers in rural areas and, finally, to work in a more professional and exclusively medical way (eschewing astrology and supplementary occupations). In considering the geographical aspects of these changes, it is crucial to understand the importance and role of medical towns. A medical town in about 1600 was to a greater or lesser extent a medical supply centre for a wide region, not just the town itself. Across the whole period three-quarters of the population living between one and six miles of the major city, Canterbury, depended on that city for medical care to the seriously ill and dying. This not only allows a reconfiguration of practitioner: population ratios, such as those for sixteenth-century Norwich devised by Margaret Pelling, but also makes it possible to examine how the importance of towns changed over time. Their hinterland-supplying roles were not static but expanding. The three-stage model for the disbursement of medical services ('urban-centred', 'urban-distributed' and 'rural-development'), demonstrates how medical practitioners' services became more evenly distributed from an initial, almost exclusively, town-centred service. Although in 1600 there possibly were some 'medically remote' spots remaining in East Kent – and undoubtedly there were in Wiltshire – it is very unlikely that by 1680 anywhere in East Kent, West Sussex or Berkshire could be described as 'medically remote', and only in rural Wiltshire did the ability to obtain medical help remain a question of status.

Just as important as the medical disbursement model are the conclusions with regard to the social background of patients. It has been demonstrated that the lower status groups in this study came to adopt medical strategies for their dying members on a level not dissimilar to that of the higher status groups. Moreover, although in the past this would be characterised as the rich employing doctors of physic and the less well-off employing 'quacks', such stereotypes are not sustainable in relation to the treatment afforded the dying. It is clear that, while some eminent physicians served only the wealthy, many formally-qualified practitioners served all, rich and poor, and, indeed, attended a wide range of less well-off dying patients at home. This strongly supports Ronald Sawyer's findings with regard to Napier's practice in Buckinghamshire and is in contrast to some previous understandings expressed on the basis of a few surviving casebooks.[1] There is also good evidence that access to physicians by lower status groups (relative to that by higher status groups) increased substantially. A similar increase is noticeable with regard to the relative accessibility by lower status groups to surgeons. This cannot simply be attributed to lower costs. There were some substantial increases in medical costs: for upper and lower status groups in all counties, costs of medical intervention doubled over the course of the seventeenth century. Attitudes were changing, over and above the financial implications of engaging a surgeon or physician.

---

[1]   See, for example, Nagy, *Popular medicine*, 32, based on the casebooks of Symcotts and Hall.

Another major finding with regard to East Kent, which has wide implications for understanding medical services, is the high proportion of practitioners attending the dying who were in some way qualified. Few historians would previously have guessed that approximately 30–40 per cent of practitioners attending the dying were diocesan licentiates. The assumption prevalent before 1960 – that most 'proper' physicians resided in London and most medical practitioners outside the capital were unqualified – has here been laid to rest. As shown in chapter 3, the number of unlicensed practitioners was a little more than the number of licentiates, but among the ranks of the 'unlicensed practitioners' are MDs and MBs. As the more detailed studies in chapter 4 make clear, before 1650 about two-thirds of identifiable practitioners were in some way 'qualified', and after the Interregnum this increased slightly, to perhaps about 75 per cent. What is interesting about the qualifications is the growing tendency to deviate from the epithets accorded to the practitioners. Despite the fact that these patients all died, more medical practitioners assisting the dying were accorded the generic high-status description 'doctor', indicating an increasing degree of respect, as well as perhaps highlighting a more general capability to deal with a range of ailments and to prescribe medicines.

The findings with regard to nursing services are hardly any less significant. First, by using the non-gender-oriented bias of the sources, it has been possible to explore quantitatively the male contribution to nursing for the first time. A mere 6 per cent of paid assistance being undertaken by men, even including the acute situations of illnesses resulting in death, suggests more confidence than before in nursing as viewed through the prism of female employment and social obligations.[2] Second, although the definition of sick-nursing in this study is exclusive of medical care, such a definition is not inappropriate. Very few female practitioners indeed are noted in these accounts in the context of advising, treating or administering physic to the dying. Furthermore, the specific examination of how frequently medicines were obtained in circumstances where no occupationally defined physician, surgeon or doctor was paid demonstrate that it was comparatively rare for nurses independently to obtain medical substances on behalf of the dying. In the late sixteenth century, when three-quarters of all interventions took the character of nursing attendance without a medical practitioner's assistance, no more than 11 per cent of these nurse-assisted families obtained a medicine from outside the household. A century later, when less than a quarter of all interventions assumed this character, no more than 39 per cent (and perhaps only 3 per cent) of these nurse-assisted families obtained medicines independently of medical practitioners. While the boundary between the remedial and the palliative is debatable – especially with regard to diet – it

---

[2] For comment on male involvement and 'acute situations' see Pelling, *Common lot*, 200–1.

would appear that only about 10 per cent of paid nursing assistance involved taking a medical initiative and obtaining medicines on behalf of the dying. Furthermore, it would appear that the bulk of paid 'nursing' care involved domestic help of a routine nature, in many cases permitting a wife to tend her husband. Finally, with regard to changes across the century, this study makes it clear that over the course of the century attending the ill person became more specialised and more clearly identifiable with occupational or semi-occupational independent mature female nurses, the evolution of the female-specific term 'nurse' permitting a comparison with the male-specific term 'doctor' by 1690.

The emphasis so far has naturally been on availability, and thus on the supply side of the economic balance. However, while the patterns of supply may well illustrate how changes in the character of medical interventions could facilitate a far broader programme of care, they do not in themselves explain why the changes took place. Nor do they explain how changes in demand manifest themselves in relation to supply. For example, the increased proportions of dying patients who were visited by their practitioners cannot be squared with a relatively unchanging number of medical practitioners without the families of dying men more frequently requesting that the practitioner come to the bedside: payments for which are a reflection of demand as much of supply. Thus, while acknowledging that supply was certainly a factor in the increased use of medicine by the dying, most probably based on the increased use of chemical medicines and a greater willingness to attend the dying, an explanation for the reasons for the changes quantified in this study must include an explanation of the changes in demand.

Medical help for the dying cannot be treated as merely another commodity. This is the problem with applying traditional economic methods to medical history: the market forces of demand and supply are two-dimensional, and what is required here is a multi-dimensional approach. Fundamental attitudes towards death and healing, as well as towards medicine, must be considered and, in particular, the perceived power of God to punish sinners with illness and, conversely, to save the penitent from death. From the evidence of seventeenth-century diaries it is abundantly clear that religious and medical strategies for coping with severe and terminal illness coexisted with and complemented one another throughout the seventeenth century. The findings of this study show that the rise of medical strategies coincided with the decline in exclusive reliance on spiritual strategies. The greatly increased volumes of metal-based medicines imported in and soon after 1600 may help further to explain this: the increased selection of medicaments available to sufferers encouraged them to try medical means of coping with medical crises, to the diminution of the exclusive use of prayer.[3] The increased use

---

[3]   The value of imports of metal-based medicines increased eightfold between 1600 and 1620: Pelling and Webster, 'Medical practitioners', 178–9; Roberts, 'Personnel and practice', pt I, 369–70; pt II, 227.

of medical assistance does not diminish the importance of religion as an element in a recovery strategy, but it strongly militates against religion or faith being the sole strategy. Indeed, it is clear that by 1700, when most of the dying obtained some medical help shortly before death, an exclusively spiritual strategy could not have been the recourse of the majority, whereas in 1600 it could, and probably was.

Broadly speaking, then, it might be said that the evidence of the probate accounts supports the widely-held belief that the advent of scientific methods challenged and ultimately reduced religious faith. This is a superficial reading of the evidence: it would be hard to argue that religion declined in importance over the course of the seventeenth century, and even harder to argue that it had declined by 1650, by which date the increase in medical assistance was well underway. Furthermore, there is ample evidence that providence remained an essential component of medical understanding long after the period 1620–50, when the first dramatic increases in medical usage took place. Indeed, religious views on death and illness probably encouraged a shift towards medical strategies. This is most clearly illustrated in a letter from Maria Thynne to her husband, dated 1608: 'Remember we are bound in conscience to maintain life as long as is possible, and though God's power can work miracles, yet we cannot build upon it that because He can, He will, for then He would not say He made herb[s] for the use of man.'[4] Herein lies the 'conflict' between perceptions of spiritual cure and medical relief. Within a spiritual context one could – and should – take medicines because they were provided by God for that purpose.

The implications of this argument are considerable. A multi-dimensional approach to medical intervention makes it possible to see the increased importation of medical substances and the spread of Paracelsian ideas in the decades either side of 1600 within a framework of expanding religious horizons. Medicines were not just an alternative to prayer, they were a supplement to prayer. The adoption of a medical strategy alongside a religious one increased the number of ways in which God's cure might be effected. This explains why medical ideas and discoveries so quickly took hold within communities: in the eyes of the dying man a new therapy was not a challenge to God's power but a blessing. Repeated decades of such blessings, however, resulted in the focus shifting from God as the provider to the therapy itself. By 1690, when the majority of people tended to choose a medical strategy to cope with fatal illness and injury, the religious framework to medical cure had ceased to dominate attitudes to treatment in the face of death. The power to affect the fate of a sick individual had been relocated, from the exclusively divine to the largely physical.

In this light a new model may be proposed for the medicalisation of serious illnesses and injuries resulting in death, and to explain how that

4   This is quoted in Houlbrooke, *Death, religion and the family*, 18–19.

medicalisation might have been fostered within the apparently non-scientific framework of religious orthodoxy. The essence of this change may be regarded as lying in the nature of the new medical ideas and substances which came into England in the last decade of the sixteenth century and the early decades of the seventeenth. Being a medical philosophy essentially composed of things, which could be regarded as substances provided by God, and which did not in itself question that the origin of healing power lay with God (unlike, for example, magic), it provided an ancillary process through which the desperate and dying could seek relief from physical suffering. This approach provides a refinement of the theory proposed by Keith Thomas in the last chapter of *Religion and the decline of magic*. Therein Thomas argued that magic weakened as people gained greater control over the environment, although he admitted that the explanation of how 'magical' systems of belief came to be seen as 'intellectually unsatisfactory' was far from clear, there being 'too many "rationalists" beforehand and too many believers afterwards'.[5] Control over the 'environment', including the landscape of disease, may well have been a contributory factor, but the process by which one belief system gives way to another should not necessarily be seen in terms of conflict. The strength of belief in spiritual physic when medical strategies to life-threatening diseases and injuries were becoming universally popular suggests rather that a religious system might have given way naturally to a scientific one through a process of accommodating scientific changes within the existing religious framework.

It is easier to account for the changes in the nature of nursing over the period in question. Expansions of medical knowledge are not necessary to explain greater confidence in the ability of nurses to deliver care, especially as a number of nursing services were of a common or domestic work nature. Also, the labour market on which nursing depended was a relatively narrowly defined one, and hardly (if at all) expanding, consisting of local residents, and, increasingly, local experienced women. Most significantly, the major changes in nursing were more or less contemporary with – or just later than – the most rapid increases in payments for medical assistance. The period 1640–60 (only partially covered by these accounts) seems to be the watershed for the terminology and activities of sick-nursing, and the apparent exclusion of maids, boys, the poor and the wider parish community from the tasks of watching and helping. At about this time the increasingly common medical approach to dealing with fatal illnesses probably affected nursing care too, so that versatile, experienced reliable people were required, who could serve sometimes for long periods of time, to the exclusion of other members of the community. Such requirements naturally would have favoured those women who were older, without young children, who could perform a wide

5   K. Thomas, *Religion and the decline of magic: studies in popular beliefs in sixteenth and seventeenth century England*, London 1971, 647.

range of household tasks and who (on the whole) did not have competing occupational commitments. But why the change? One explanation may be the spread of the task of administering medicines provided by physicians and doctors to the sick, and helping to present an ordered household for a physician or surgeon to attend. Another explanation may be that local women had an almost exclusive control over the care of those suffering from contagious diseases and, in the period 1620–60 (when the care process was increasingly seen in terms of medicinal intervention), female care of the contagious sick also became more medicinal. It is probable that both of these aspects resulted in an increased medical role for the small number of women who specialised in the care of the dying. It might be argued that older women found nursing one of the few available occupational specialisms open to them, as it required no formal qualifications, did not normally require long-distance travel, and yet was an area of work in which a woman could acquire a local reputation as a helper and as an instrument of God's healing work, albeit with some negative connotations in the cities.

A lot more work needs to be done in this area. Investigations into the causes of the changes noted in this study almost certainly cannot be conducted using quantitative methods but require a thorough examination of the developing expectations of medicine and nursing among the varying constituencies that are represented in these accounts: the very old and decrepit, the infected, the insane and the injured. Here they are practically inseparable. It is likely, however, that a separation of the old from the diseased and injured would reveal different patterns of treatment and nursing care. The attempt to do this for the contagious in chapter 6 demonstrated that this group displays patterns of its own with regard to both medical assistance and nursing, distinct from the collective gamut of the dying. Further work on the distinction between palliative and remedial care amongst nurses and helpers especially would be useful, and may be possible to a certain extent using the instances in these records where nurses and helpers seem to have been involved in taking medical initiatives. Closer examinations of aspects of this study which here have been treated generally and quantitatively will undoubtedly pay dividends to the student more interested in the medical than the social implications of medicalisation. The challenge is to examine how the changes here reflect the intellectual developments of the early seventeenth century; there is an undoubted opportunity for someone to explore how, in East Kent, increased frequency of medical care to the dying might reflect varying levels of practitioner knowledge and confidence in practitioners' expertise, and greater varieties of available medicines.

The tripartite system has been shown to be a loose description of medical care. From the frequency with which practitioners swapped or assumed new identities to the taking of medical initiatives by nurses, every element is open to question. This should not be a surprise, for significant changes in the ways people behaved on behalf of their seriously ill and dying relatives have been charted, and if there are tensions and contradictions within such a system, these are merely symptomatic of the rapidity with which that system was evolving. By the end of this period the strategy of seeking the help of an appropriate medical specialist for a seriously ill or dying individual, and paying for experienced nurses to minister to him in his last sickness, is recognisable and perhaps correctly described as modern. At the start of the period such palliative assistance was normally inexpert and community-led; there was little occupational medical expertise obtained on behalf of the patient, and there was a much stronger religious context to the final days of a man's life. Whether this fundamental change amounts to the medicalisation of society as a whole, or only a part of it, is a subject which will exercise minds in the future, but there is no doubt that the advent of new medicines allowed a totally new perspective on ill-health. Through the rapid economic distribution of medical substances and the medical men who could administer them, fundamental changes took place in the understanding and handling of severe illness, in that the fate of a severely ill patient was increasingly seen to be a matter for human – not divine – intervention. The importance of this in the social history of medicine cannot be overestimated, and in terms of general social history it is hardly any less significant. In attempting to understand the key differences between life in England before and after the mid-seventeenth century, the relocation of human well-being from the predominantly divine to the predominantly physical should be considered one of the most profound revolutions that society has ever experienced.

Medical Indices for East Kent, West Sussex, Berkshire and Wiltshire

1. East Kent

	Urban A, B, R	Urban C, D, S	1–6 miles A, B, R	1–6 miles C, D, S
A: 1570–99	12/119	38/565	20/249	48/1385
B: 1600–49	125/562	214/1719	146/1118	219/3259
C: 1660–89	177/495	192/701	241/862	242/1130
D: 1690–1719	42/91	33/69	125/238	41/96
Increase				
D/A	4.6	7.1	6.5	12.3
C/A	3.6	4.1	3.5	6.2
C/B	1.6	2.2	2.1	3.2

Note: Status groups A, B, C, D (men), and R, S (women) are as outlined in chapter 1.

2. West Sussex

	Urban A, B, R	Urban C, D, S	1–6 miles A, B, R	1–6 miles C, D, S
B: 1600–49	6/38	9/86	18/191	13/344
C: 1660–89	10/31	11/30	32/161	14/107
Increase				
C/B	[2.0]	[3.5]	2.1	3.5

3. Berkshire

	Urban A, B, R	Urban C, D, S	1–6 miles A, B, R	1–6 miles C, D, S
B: 1600–49	4/50	24/196	11/158	23/555
C: 1660–89	7/40	3/51	20/143	17/154
Increase				
C/B	[2.2]	[0.5]	2.0	2.7

213

4. Wiltshire

	Urban A, B, R	Urban C, D, S	1–6 miles A, B, R	1–6 miles C, D, S
B: 1600–49	1/23	3/128	5/70	8/288
C: 1660–89	8/29	7/60	10/69	2/73
Increase				
C/B	[6.3]	5.0	2.0	1.0

Square brackets relate to indices calculated on periods with fewer than fifty accounts for the status group in that county.

Bibliography

Unpublished primary sources

Chichester, West Sussex Record Office
EpI/33 Consistory court of the archdeaconry of Chichester: probate accounts, 1572–1710
EpIII/9; EpIV/10 Peculiar court of the dean of Chichester: probate accounts, 1599–1616, 1610–84

Exeter, Devon Record Office
Chanter 41–9 Act books of the diocese of Exeter, 1568–97, 1610–46, 1661–1734
Moger II/surgeons' licences: petitions for medical licences of the diocese of Exeter

London, Wellcome Trust Library
MSS 5343–7 A. W. G. Haggis, typescript list of medical licentiates

Maidstone, Centre for Kentish Studies
PRC 1/1–18 Archdeaconry court of the diocese of Canterbury: probate accounts, 1569–1700
PRC 2/1–42 Archdeaconry court of the diocese of Canterbury: probate accounts, 1600–1728
PRC 21/1–17 Consistory court of the diocese of Canterbury: probate accounts, 1569–1605
PRC 20/1–13 Consistory court of the diocese of Canterbury: probate accounts, 1605–91
PRC 19/1–6 Consistory court of the diocese of Canterbury: probate accounts, 1635–1729
Corpe, S., 'A register of the freemen of Canterbury', unpublished typescripts, 1550–1650, 1650–1700, 1700–50

Reading, Berkshire Record Office
D/A1/35–225 Archdeaconry court of Berkshire: probate accounts, 1564–1725
D/A2/C5-C25 Archdeaconry court of Berkshire: probate accounts, 1564–87
D/A3/2–4 Peculiar court of the dean of Sarum: probate accounts, 1666–93

Trowbridge, Wiltshire and Swindon Record Office
Miscellaneous wills bk 6: Peculiar court of Trowbridge: probate account, 1635
P1 Consistory court of the diocese of Sarum: probate accounts, 1595–1738
P2 Archdeaconry court of Sarum: probate accounts, 1576–1704
P3 Archdeaconry court of Wiltshire: probate accounts, 1600–1713
P4 Peculiar court of the subdean of Sarum: probate accounts, 1612–1702
P5 Peculiar court of the dean of Sarum: probate accounts, 1585–1693

Chantor Sarum Bundle 2, 4 9, 10 Peculiar court of the precentor of Sarum: probate accounts, 1609–81
Peculiar court of the dean and canons of Windsor: probate accounts, 1641–77
Peculiar court of the dean and chapter of Sarum: probate accounts, 1606–81
Peculiar court of the Lord Warden of Savernake Forest: probate accounts
Peculiar court of the perpetual vicar of Corsham: probate accounts, 1618–77
Peculiar court of the prebendary of Bishopstone: probate accounts, 1600–30
Peculiar court of the prebendary of Chute and Chisenbury: probate account, 1597
Peculiar court of the prebendary of Coombe and Harnham: probate account, 1696
Peculiar court of the prebendary of Durnford: probate account, 1628
Peculiar court of the prebendary of Highworth: probate accounts, 1596–1675
Peculiar court of the prebendary of Lyme Regis and Halstock: probate account, 1627
Peculiar court of the prebendary of Netheravon: probate account, 1635
Peculiar court of the treasurer of Sarum: probate accounts, 1594–1689

Published primary sources

Administrations and inventories of the archdeaconry of Northampton (now preserved in the County Record Office at Northampton), ed. C. Baggott (British Record Society Ltd, Index Library xcii, 1980)

Berkshire probate accounts, 1583–1712, ed. I. Mortimer (Berkshire Record Society iv, 1999)

Canterbury licences (general), 1568–1646, ed. A. J. Willis, Chichester 1972

The Compton Census of 1676: a critical edition, ed. A. Whiteham (British Academy, Records of Social and Economic History x, 1986)

Exeter freemen, 1266–1967, ed. M. M. Rowe and A. M. Jackson (Devon and Cornwall Record Society e.s. i, 1973)

A Hampshire miscellany, II: Laymen's licences of the diocese of Winchester, 1675–1834, ed. A. J. Willis, Folkestone 1964

Index to the probate accounts of England and Wales, A-J, ed. P. Spufford (British Record Society Ltd, Index Library cxii, 1999)

The register of Walter Stapledon, bishop of Exeter, ed. F. C. Hingeston Randolph, Exeter 1892

The roll of the Royal College of Physicians of London compiled from the annals of the college and from other authentic sources, ed. W. Munk, London 1861

A seventeenth century doctor and his patients: John Symcotts, 1592–1662, ed. F. N. L. Poynter and W. J. Bishop (Bedfordshire Historical Record Society xxxi, 1951)

Seventeenth century economic documents, ed. J. Thirsk and J. P. Cooper, Oxford 1972

Stockport probate records, 1620–1650, ed. C. B. Phillips and J. H. Smith (Record Society of Lancashire and Cheshire cxxxi, 1992)

Tradesmen in early Stuart Wiltshire, ed. N. J. Williams (Wiltshire Archaeological and Natural History Society, 1960)

BIBLIOGRAPHY

Reference works

Anon., A physicall dictionary, London 1657
Bartholomews gazetteer, 9th edn, London 1943, repr. 1966
Blancard, S., A physical dictionary; in which all the terms relating either to anatomy, chirugery, pharmacy, or chymistry, are very accurately explain'd, London 1684
Blount, T., Glossographia, 2nd edn, London 1661
Coles, E., An English dictionary, 2nd edn, London 1685
Kellys directory of Kent, London 1939
Lewis, S., Topographical dictionary of England, 7th edn, London 1849
Phillips, E., A new world of English words, 1st edn, London 1657
Ruffhead, O., Statutes at large, London 1786
Venn, J., Alumni cantabrigienses, pt 1, Cambridge 1922–7

Secondary sources

Abel-Smith, B., A history of the nursing profession, London 1960
Ariès, P. (trans. H. Weaver), The hour of our death, Oxford 1991
Arkell, T., 'A method for estimating population totals from the Compton Census returns', in K. Schurer and T. Arkell (eds), Surveying the people: the interpretation and use of document sources for the study of population in the later seventeenth century, Oxford 1992, 97–116
—— 'Interpreting probate inventories', in Arkell, Evans and Goose, When death us do part, 72–102
—— 'The probate process', in Arkell, Evans and Goose, When death us do part, 3–13
—— N. Evans and N. Goose (eds), When death us do part, Oxford 2000
Barry, J., 'Piety and the patient: medicine and religion in eighteenth century Bristol', in Porter, Patients and practitioners, 145–76
—— 'Population distribution and growth in the early modern period', in R. Kain and W. Ravenhill (eds), Historical atlas of south-west England, Exeter 1999, 116–17
—— 'South-west', in Clark, The Cambridge urban history of Britain, ii. 67–92
Beaufort, D. A., 'The medical practitioners of western Sussex in the early modern period: a preliminary survey' (Sussex Archaeological Collections cxxxi, 1993), 139–51
Beier, L. McC., Sufferers and healers, London 1987
—— 'The good death', in Houlbrooke, Death, ritual, and bereavement, 43–61
Bishop, W. J., 'Transport and the doctor in Great Britain', Bulletin of the History of Medicine xxii (1948), 427–39
Bowden, P. (ed.), Chapters from the agrarian history of England and Wales, 1500–1750, I: Economic change: prices, wages, profits and rents, 1500–1750, Cambridge 1990
Bower, J., 'Probate accounts as a source for Kentish early modern economic and social history', Archaeologia Cantiana cix (1991), 51–62
—— Probate accounts (Historical Association, Short Guides to Records xxxiv, 1994)

—— 'Kent towns, 1540–1640', in M. Zell (ed.), *Early modern Kent, 1540–1640*, Woodbridge 2000, 141–76

Brandon, P. and B. Short, *The south east from AD 1000*, London 1990

Bullough, V. and B. Bullough, *The care of the sick: the emergence of modern nursing*, London 1979

Burnby, J. G. L., *A study of the English apothecary from 1660–1760* (Supplement to *Medical History* iii, 1983)

Chalklin, C. W., *Seventeenth century Kent: a social and economic history*, London 1965

Clark, A. (ed. and intro. A. L. Erickson), *Working life of women in the seventeenth century*, London 1992

Clark, P. (ed.), *The Cambridge urban history of Britain*, II: *1540–1840*, Cambridge 2000

Cox, J. and N. Cox, 'Probate, 1500–1800: a system in transition', in Arkell, Evans and Goose, *When death us do part*, 14–37

Cressy, D., *Birth, marriage and death: ritual, religion, and the life-cycle in Tudor and Stuart England*, Oxford 1997

Dils, J., 'Berkshire towns, 1500–1700', in J. Dils (ed.), *An historical map of Berkshire* (Berkshire Record Society, 1998), 50–1

Dobson, M., *Contours of death and disease in early modern England*, Cambridge 1997

Dock, L. and I. Stewart, *A short history of nursing from the earliest times to the present day*, 4th edn, New York 1938

Ehrenreich, B. and D. English, *Witches, midwives and nurses: a history of women healers*, New York 1973

Erickson, A. L., 'An introduction to probate accounts', in G. Martin and P. Spufford, *The records of the nation*, Woodbridge 1990, 273–86

—— *Women and property in early modern England*, London 1993

—— 'Using probate accounts', in Arkell, Evans and Goose, *When death us do part*, 103–19

Evenden, D. (née Nagy), 'Mothers and their midwives in seventeenth-century London', in Marland, *Art of midwifery*, 9–26

—— *The midwives of seventeenth century London*, Cambridge 2000

Everitt, A., 'Market towns, c.1500–1640', in J. Thirsk (ed.), *The agrarian history of England and Wales*, iv, Cambridge 1967, 466–589

Gittings, C., *Death, burial and the individual in early modern England*, London 1984

—— 'Probate accounts: a neglected source', *The Local Historian* (May 1991), 51–9

Grell, O. P. and A. Cunningham (eds), *Medicine and the Reformation*, London 1993

Guy, J., 'The episcopal licensing of physicians, surgeons and midwives', *Bulletin of the History of Medicine* lvi (1982), 528–42

Harley, D., 'Provincial midwives in England: Lancashire and Cheshire, 1660–1760', in Marland, *Art of midwifery*, 27–48

—— 'Spiritual physic, providence and English medicine', in Grell and Cunningham, *Medicine and the Reformation*, 101–17

—— 'Bred up in the study of that faculty: licensed physicians in north-west England, 1660–1760', *Medical History* xxxviii (1994), 398–420

Hess, A. G., 'Midwifery practice among the Quakers in southern rural England in the late 17th century', in Marland, Art of midwifery, 49–76

Holmes, G., Augustan England: professions, state and society, 1680–1730, London 1982

Houlbrooke, R. (ed.), Death, ritual, and bereavement, London 1989

—— Death, religion and the family in England, 1480–1750, Oxford 1998

Hull, F., Guide to the Kent County Archives Office, Maidstone 1958

James, R. R., 'Licences to practise medicine and surgery issued by the archbishops of Canterbury, 1580–1775', Janus xli (1937), 97–106

—— 'The earliest list of surgeons to be licensed', Janus xli (1937), 255–60

King, S. and A. Weaver, 'Lives in many hands: the medical landscape in Lancashire, 1700–1820', Medical History xlv (2000), 173–200

Lane, J., 'The medical practitioners of provincial England', Medical History xxviii (1984), 353–71

—— The social history of medicine, London 2001

Laslett, P., The world we have lost further explored, 3rd edn, London 1983; 2000

Laurence, A., Women in England, 1500–1760, London 1994

Loudon, I., Medical care and the general practitioner, 1750–1850, Oxford 1987

—— 'Medical practitioners, 1750–1850, and the period of medical reform in Britain', in Wear, Medicine in society, 219–48

McConaghey, R. M. S., 'The history of rural medical practice', in Poynter, Medical practice in Britain, 117–43

MacDonald, M., Mystical Bedlam: madness, medicine and history in seventeenth century England, Cambridge 1981

Macfarlane, A., The origins of English individualism, Oxford 1978

Maggs, C., The origins of general nursing, London 1983

Marland, H. (ed.), The art of midwifery: early modern midwives in Europe, London 1993

Matthews, L. G., History of pharmacy in Britain, Edinburgh 1962

—— 'Spicers and apothecaries in the city of Canterbury', Medical History ix (1965), 289–91

Mendelson, S. and P. Crawford, Women in early modern England, Oxford 1998

Mortimer, I., 'Diocesan licensing and medical practitioners in south-west England, 1660–1780', Medical History xlviii (2004), 49–68

—— 'Index of medical licentiates, applicants, referees and examiners in the diocese of Exeter, 1568–1783', Transactions of the Devonshire Association cxxxvi (2004), 99–134

—— 'The triumph of the doctors: medical assistance to the dying, c.1570–1720', Transactions of the Royal Historical Society 6th ser. xv (2005), 97–116

—— 'A directory of medical personnel qualified and practising in the diocese of Canterbury, c.1560–1730', Archaeologia Cantiana cxxvi (2006), 135–69

—— 'Why were probate accounts made? Methodological issues concerning the historical use of administrators' and executors' accounts', Archives xxxi (2006), 2–17

Muldrew, C., 'Hard food for Midas: cash and its social value in early modern England', Past and Present clxx (2001), 78–120.

Nagy, D. Popular medicine in seventeenth century England, Bowling Green 1988

O'Day, R., Professions in early modern England, London 2000

Overton, M., 'Prices from probate inventories', in Arkell, Evans and Goose, *When death us do part*, 120–43

Pelling, M., 'Tradition and diversity: medical practice in Norwich, 1550–1640', in Instituto Nazionale de Studi sul Rinascimento, *Scienze credenze occulte livelli di cultura*, Florence 1982, 159–71

—— 'Apothecaries and other medical practitioners in Norwich around 1600', *Pharmaceutical Historian* xiii (1983), 5–8

—— *The common lot*, London 1998

—— *Medical conflicts in early modern London: patronage, physicians, and irregular practitioners, 1550–1640*, Oxford 2003

—— and C. Webster, 'Medical practitioners', in Webster, *Health, medicine and morality*, 165–236

—— and R. M. Smith (eds), *Life, death and the elderly: historical perspectives*, London 1991

Pollock, L., *With faith and physic: the life of a Tudor gentlewoman, Lady Grace Mildmay, 1552–1620*, London 1993

Porter, D. and R. Porter, *Patient's progress: doctors and doctoring in eighteenth-century England*, Oxford 1989

Porter, R., *Disease, medicine and society in England, 1550–1860*, London 1987

—— 'Death and the doctors in Georgian England', in Houlbrooke, *Death, ritual and bereavement*, 77–94

—— 'The patient in England, c. 1660–1800', in Wear, *Medicine in society*, 91–118

—— (ed.), *Patients and practitioners: lay perceptions of medicine in pre-industrial society*, Cambridge 1985

—— and D. Porter, *In sickness and in health*, London 1988

Poynter, F. N. L. (ed.), *The evolution of medical practice in Britain*, London 1961

Raach, J., *A directory of English country physicians, 1603–1643*, London 1962

Roberts, R. S., 'The personnel and practice of medicine in Tudor and Stuart England: part 1: the provinces', *Medical History* vi (1962), 363–82

—— 'The personnel and practice of medicine in Tudor and Stuart England: part 2: London', *Medical History* viii (1964), 217–34

Rowse, A. L., *Simon Forman: sex and society in Shakespeare's age*, London 1974

Sharpe, P., *Women's work: the English experience, 1650–1914*, London 1998

Slack, P., 'Poverty and politics in Salisbury, 1597–1666', in P. Clark and P. Slack (eds), *Crisis and order in English towns, 1500–1700*, London 1972, 164–203

—— 'Mirrors of health and treasures of poor men: the use of the vernacular medical literature of Tudor England', in Webster, *Health, medicine and mortality*, 9–60

—— *Impact of plague in Tudor and Stuart England*, London 1985

Spufford, M., *The great reclothing of rural England*, London 1984

—— 'The limitations of the probate inventory', in J. Chartres and D. Hey (eds), *English rural society, 1500–1800*, London 1990, 139–74

Spufford, P., 'Long term rural credit in sixteenth and seventeenth century England: the evidence of probate accounts', in Arkell, Evans and Goose, *When death us do part*, 213–28

Tarver, A., 'Understanding probate accounts and their generation in the post-Restoration diocese of Lichfield and Coventry to 1700', in Arkell, Evans and Goose, *When death us do part*, 229–54

Thomas, K., *Religion and the decline of magic: studies in popular beliefs in sixteenth and seventeenth century England*, London 1971

Thompson, G. S., *Life in a noble household*, London 1937

Traister, B. H., *The notorious astrological physician of London: works and days of Simon Forman*, Chicago 2001

Vaisey, D., 'Probate inventories and provincial retailers in the seventeenth century', in P. Riden (ed.), *Probate records and the local community*, Gloucester 1985, 91–112

Versluysen, M., 'Old wives' tales? Women healers in English history', in C. Davies (ed.), *Rewriting nursing history*, London 1980, 175–99

Vigarello, G. (trans. J. Birrell), *Concepts of cleanliness: changing attitudes in France since the Middle Ages*, Cambridge 1988

Wear, A., 'Puritan perceptions of illness in seventeenth century England', in Porter, *Patients and practitioners*, 55–100

—— 'Caring for the sick poor in St Bartholomew Exchange, 1580–1676', in R. Porter and W. Bynum (eds), *Living and dying in London* (Supplement to *Medical History* xi, 1991), 41–60

—— 'Making sense of health and the environment in early modern England', in Wear, *Medicine in society*, 119–48

—— 'Medical practice in late seventeenth- and early eighteenth-century England: continuity and union', in Grell and Cunningham, *Medicine and the Reformation*, 294–320

—— 'Religious beliefs and medicine in early modern England', in H. Marland and M. Pelling (eds), *The task of healing*, Rotterdam 1996, 146–69

—— (ed.), *Medicine in society*, Cambridge 1992

Webster, C. (ed.), *Health, medicine and morality in the sixteenth century*, Cambridge 1979

Williams, N. J., *Tradesmen in Early Stuart Wiltshire*, Devizes 1960

Wilson, P. K., *Surgery, skin and syphilis*, Amsterdam, Atlanta 1999

Wrigley, E. A. and R. Schofield, *The population history of England, 1841–1871*, London 1981

Wyman, A. L., 'The surgeoness: the female practitioner of surgery, 1400–1800', *Medical History* xxviii (1984), 22–41

Unpublished dissertations

Mortimer, I., 'Medical assistance to the dying in provincial southern England, c.1570–1720', PhD, Exeter 2004

Sawyer, R., 'Patients, healers and disease in the south east Midlands, 1597–1634', PhD, Wisconsin–Madison 1985

Index

Ingram Content Group UK Ltd.
Milton Keynes UK
UKHW020019100323
418330UK00006B/363